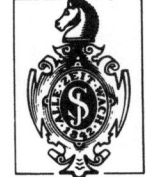

P. D. Coleridge Smith · J. H. Scurr (Eds.)

Microcomputers in Medicine

With 76 Figures

Springer-Verlag
Berlin Heidelberg GmbH

P. D. Coleridge Smith, MA, BM, FRCS
Senior Lecturer in Surgical Science, Department of Surgical Studies,
University College and Middlesex School of Medicine, Mortimer
Street, London W1N 8AA, UK.

J. H. Scurr, BSc, FRCS
Senior Lecturer in Surgery and Honorary Consultant Surgeon,
Department of Surgical Studies, University College and Middlesex
School of Medicine, Mortimer Street, London W1N 8AA, UK.

ISBN 978-1-4471-1615-8   ISBN 978-1-4471-1613-4 (eBook)
DOI 10.1007/978-1-4471-1613-4

British Library Cataloguing in Publication Data
Coleridge Smith, P.D. (Philip David), 1953–
Microcomputers in medicine.
1. Medicine. Applications of microcomputer systems
I. Title   II. Scurr, J.H. (John Henry), 1947–
610'.28'5416

Library of Congress Cataloging-in-Publication Data
Microcomputers in medicine / P. D. Coleridge Smith and J. H. Scurr (eds.).
     p.   cm.
   Based on the proceedings of the Fourth Medical Microcomputer Workshop held at
the Middlesex Hospital Medical School on Sept. 3–5, 1986.
   Includes bibliographies and index.

   1. Medicine—Data processing—Congresses. 2 Microcomputers—Congresses. I.
Coleridge Smith, P.D. (Philip David), 1953–   . II. Scurr, J. H. (John Henry),
1947–   . III. Medical Microcomputer Workshop (4th : 1986 : Middlesex
Hospital Medical School) IV. Title: Microcomputers in medicine
[DNLM: 1. Automatic Data Processing. 2. Computers. W 26.5 M62594 1986]
R858.A2M5 1988 610'.285416—dc 19 DNLM/DLC for Library of Congress 88–
4480 CIP

Filmset by Wilmaset, Birkenhead, Merseyside
Printed at the University Printing House, Oxford

2128/3916-543210

Preface

This book is based on the proceedings of the fourth Medical Microcomputer Workshop held at the Middlesex Hospital Medical School on 3–5 September 1986. The workshop was attended by clinicians and computer scientists with an interest in applying computer technology to current medical practice. The problems ranged from audit and patient management through to the more complex applications of data analysis obtained from current diagnostic techniques.

The choice of microcomputers has never been greater with low cost making them readily available. A single microcomputer has limitations in clinical practice and the use of networks for multi-user tasks has expanded its capability but increased the complexity both in terms of hardware and the software needed to run it. Although comprehensive commercial packages are available, none of these are entirely suitable for medical applications without modification. Many of the chapters presented in this book describe the problems encountered and the solutions achieved by configuring and modifying applications software.

The most widely used microcomputer application in medicine is for clinical audit. A number of commercially available systems have been developed but variations in local practice have limited their introduction. There is still no general agreement on which data should be recorded and how they should be used. The current systems for encoding data have their limitations, particularly in research applications when the precision of these codes is poor. Most systems still require dedicated medical staff to enter the data to avoid errors, but the development of automatic data entry systems may decrease the workload and increase efficiency.

This book contains chapters describing the development of audit techniques, their application, problems encountered and the solutions achieved. The experience of the contributors in solving these problems will be invaluable to any clinician intending to develop his own audit system and will allow objective evaluation of commercial systems.

Measurement techniques in medicine are increasing in complexity. The use of microcomputers speeds data analysis and allows storage of data for subsequent processing and report generation. Contributors to this book describe several applications in the field of clinical measurement. These applications may be used directly or, with modification, may be applied to similar problems.

The development of microcomputer systems has an important educational role. This role is not only in the development of computer software but also in teaching medicine. One example of this is the development of software to simulate medical emergencies described in this book.

Department of Surgical Studies   P. D. Coleridge Smith
The Middlesex Hospital, London W1   J. H. Scurr
September 1987

Contents

Contributors

D. Barnard
Orthodontic Department, Queen Alexandra Hospital, Cosham, Portsmouth, Hants, UK

D. J. Birnie
Orthodontic Department, Queen Alexandra Hospital, Cosham, Portsmouth, Hants, UK

D. Bryce
The Faculty of Medicine Computing Unit, Ninewells Hospital and Medical School, Dundee, UK

P. D. Coleridge Smith
Department of Surgical Studies, The Middlesex Hospital, London, UK

W. A. Corbett
Department of Surgery, Royal Liverpool Hospital, University of Liverpool, Liverpool, UK

J. R. Coughlan
Department of Surgery, Royal Liverpool Hospital, University of Liverpool, Liverpool, UK

D. C. Dunn
Department of Surgery, Addenbrooke's Hospital, Cambridge, UK

P. R. Edwards
Department of Surgery, Royal Liverpool Hospital, University of Liverpool, Liverpool, UK

M. C. Fairhurst
Electronic Engineering Laboratories, University of Kent,
Canterbury, Kent, UK

N. W. T. Harradine
University of Bristol Dental School, Lower Maudlin Street, Bristol,
UK

J. D. Holdsworth
Department of Surgery, Ashington Hospital, Northumberland, UK

S. W. Kelly
Electronic Engineering Laboratories, University of Kent,
Canterbury, Kent, UK

S. J. Nixon
Department of Surgery, The Royal Infirmary, Edinburgh, UK

J. H. Scurr
Department of Surgical Studies, The Middlesex Hospital, London,
UK

S. Shami
Department of Surgery, Wexham Park Hospital, Slough, UK

J. L. Shearer
The Faculty of Medicine Computing Unit, Ninewells Hospital and
Medical School, Dundee, UK

R. Shields
Department of Surgery, Royal Liverpool Hospital, University of
Liverpool, Liverpool, UK

S. L. Smith
Electronic Engineering Laboratories, University of Kent,
Canterbury, Kent, UK

S. Stock
Department of Surgery, Newcastle General Hospital,
Newcastle-upon-Tyne, UK

M. J. Taylor
Department of Computer Science, University of Liverpool,
Liverpool, UK

M. A. Walker
The Faculty of Medicine Computing Unit, Ninewells Hospital and
Medical School, Dundee, UK

N. Wynne-Carter
The Faculty of Medicine Computing Unit, Ninewells Hospital and
Medical School, Dundee, UK

1 A Generalised Approach to Clinical Audit, Patient Management and Research

N. Wynne-Carter, M.A. Walker, D. Bryce and J.L. Shearer

Introduction. Taking the Generalised or Parametric Approach to Software Design and the Transition from Minicomputer to Networked and Stand-alone Microcomputers.

The Faculty of Medicine Computing Unit (FMCU) in Dundee has evolved within a hospital and medical school environment over the last ten years, growing out of a team of computer professionals built up around the automation of diagnostic laboratory data management. In recent years the team has been augmented by the complementary infusion of clinicians who have trained in computing skills within the Unit under the sponsorship of the Scottish Home and Health Department.

The parametric approach to systems design was taken in the early seventies with a remit to create a laboratory data management system which could not only adapt to changing requirements over its active life span but also be transferred to other laboratories without the need for re-programming for local differences [1,2]. That system has vindicated the approach in so much as it still thrives after 12 years' use and evolution in three Scottish Health Boards and was taken as a model for the original Phoenix laboratory system [3] from which many of the current commercial systems were derived.

The FMCU was formed when a minicomputer was purchased to serve the wider requirements of the medical school not catered for by remote access to the facilities of the main-frame computer on the university campus some miles distant. At that time the even more distant central health board computer department appeared unable adequately to respond to the expectations of the more forward-looking clinicians who began to look to computers for the collection and analysis of clinically orientated information for audit and research study purposes.

It was soon clear that the common theme to the requests made of the FMCU was to set up data collection systems with a view to subsequent analysis. Without the resources to create new software for each client it was decided to invest once in the development of a set of facilities which could be used without the need for re-programming for each application.

Though now a well-established concept for business applications it was then novel to remove the definition of record structures out of the software into separate configuration files created with a conversational application generation package. By reference to these files generalised data input, update and maintenance facilities were produced for the recording and indexing of records for the appropriate study. The nature of the proformas which were used to collect the clinical information called for great flexibility in the data types which were needed conveniently to record the mix of numerical and non-numerical data with many responses not relevant to particular patients. The data coding stage, commonly used at that time, was eliminated by the inclusion of configurable validation checks and on-line expansion of abbreviations. This made for an accurate and friendly conversational data-input mechanism. However the mechanism used for data analysis and presentation was not ideal. A simple language was devised which incorporated commands to access and manipulate the record structure described above. In this language some general-purpose statistical, graphical and analytical facilities were produced but all too frequently it was necessary to modify and extend them and to write special ones to provide the kinds of technique required by each user, who was therefore still too dependent upon us.

With the life span of our minicomputer drawing to a close and the dearth of university funds it was unlikely that we could replace it with another. At that time, some 3 or 4 years ago, it became possible to network microcomputers so that they could share expensive resources such as hard discs and other peripherals. With a local area network it would be possible to build up new computing facilities progressively, allowing user departments to contribute their own microcomputers from diverse funds whilst retaining the support and facilities of the FMCU.

We had some experience of networking having established a closed network linking our laboratory, ward and other minicomputers with serial connections. Terminal "patch-through" and file transfer were provided. The value of such facilities was really only appreciated by the users when the networking had to be withdrawn on the introduction of dissimilar machines replacing the first generation systems which all utilised the same locally-developed systems software still retained for the laboratory machines.

After taking advice we eventually settled on the Corvus Omninet network and more significantly adopted the UCSD P-system for software development. The P-system is a program development and run-time environment which supports the compilation, linking and debugging of software written in a variety of high and low level languages. At run-time an interpreter is used which operates on a very compact target language, the p(seudo) machine [4]. The interpreter is much faster than those operating on source code as was common with most BASIC systems, and the advantage was the transferability between machine types. The

UCSD PASCAL language was also chosen in preference to BASIC for its in-built structure and good string manipulation facilities.

The initial network (Fig. 1.1) was based upon Apple II micros with which a number of software developments were begun. During this time the demand for clinical data storage and analysis continued to increase. After a fruitless search for a suitable proprietary package to cope with this requirement and to take over the data storage and analysis commitments supported with our minicomputer software described earlier it was reluctantly decided to embark yet again upon an ambitious development to transfer the facilities to the micro environment and to upgrade the existing utilities. With a strong accent upon deriving clinical research feedback and patient recall facilities a powerful package began to emerge. Numerical statistical facilities and non-numerical tabulations were incorporated which could be set up conversationally finally removing the need for subsequent programmer support. By the time it was becoming clear that the Apple II generation of machine was unlikely to have sufficient capacity and speed to be viable in service, the 16-bit generation of micros emerged as our salvation. The P-system enabled us to transfer our software up to the IBM PC and similar machines now using a standard MSDOS-hosted version.

The wider uses of these facilities now growing into a comprehensive package were soon utilised for a wide variety of applications each of which could quickly be set up for each user. A detailed description of the package christened Craft and some of its applications follows in the next two sections [6].

The logical progression of our developments was coming to fruition. Most of the long-term data sets held on the minicomputer were transferred to the networked micros using Craft joining the newly established ones all using the

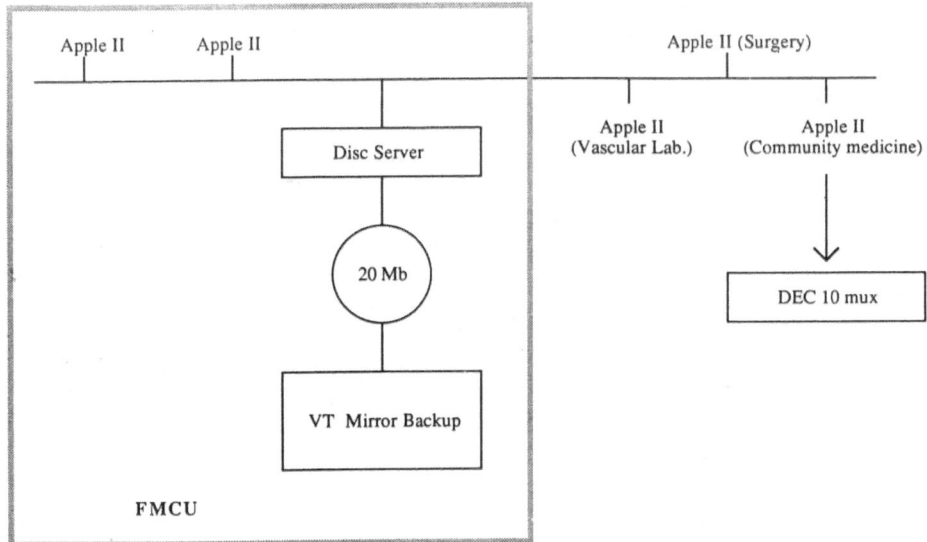

Fig. 1.1. First Omninet hardware.

Craft software. The final and largest data set which is ongoing has over 7 years of data relating to breast disease following up all malignant cases. This remains to be transferred soon.

The advantage of users attaching their micros to the Omninet network was access to substantial disc storage automatically backed-up each night to magnetic tape. In addition the maintenance of software updates is simplified by the sharing of object code.

The advent of word processing requirements has also brought new users on to the network. Some departments now have many machines attached and professors, their secretaries and other staff members share draft and laser quality printing facilities. Figure 1.2 shows the extent to which the network has now grown.

The most recent reductions in the cost of integral hard discs of substantial storage capacities now makes it possible for many users to stand alone. They do however need to perform their own back-up procedures to floppy discs or streamer tapes. This development is however perhaps a blessing as with ever-tightening university resources our network disc capacities are struggling to keep pace with the growth in demand.

The next step should be to upgrade our disc-server style networking to a file-server based system when resources permit. This more advanced network topology managed by software such as the Novell Netware [5] makes better use of the transport layer for which we can retain our Omninet equipment by adding file server micro(s), but more importantly under MSDOS version 3 it offers proper multi-user file and record protection, message broadcasting, electronic mail and the opportunity to add gateways into other networks such as the X25 main campus switches. Then we will have a true local area network.

The Craft System

Clinical Data Retrieval and Follow-up Template

For several years there has been a growing demand for an inexpensive microcomputer-based software package which would enable clinicians to collect, maintain and analyse medical data in a variety of situations such as disease registers, research projects and patient management situations, including shared care schemes. Although there are a number of comprehensive database packages available commercially, these are aimed mainly at the business world and hence are not ideally suited to the clinical situation. In general these packages have very limited facilities for dealing with and analysing non-numerical information. The origins of Craft's development were described in the previous section. The system which has emerged is now described in some detail.

System Structure

The system has been structured around the concept of a control file in which each subject registered with an application has one control record. This unique

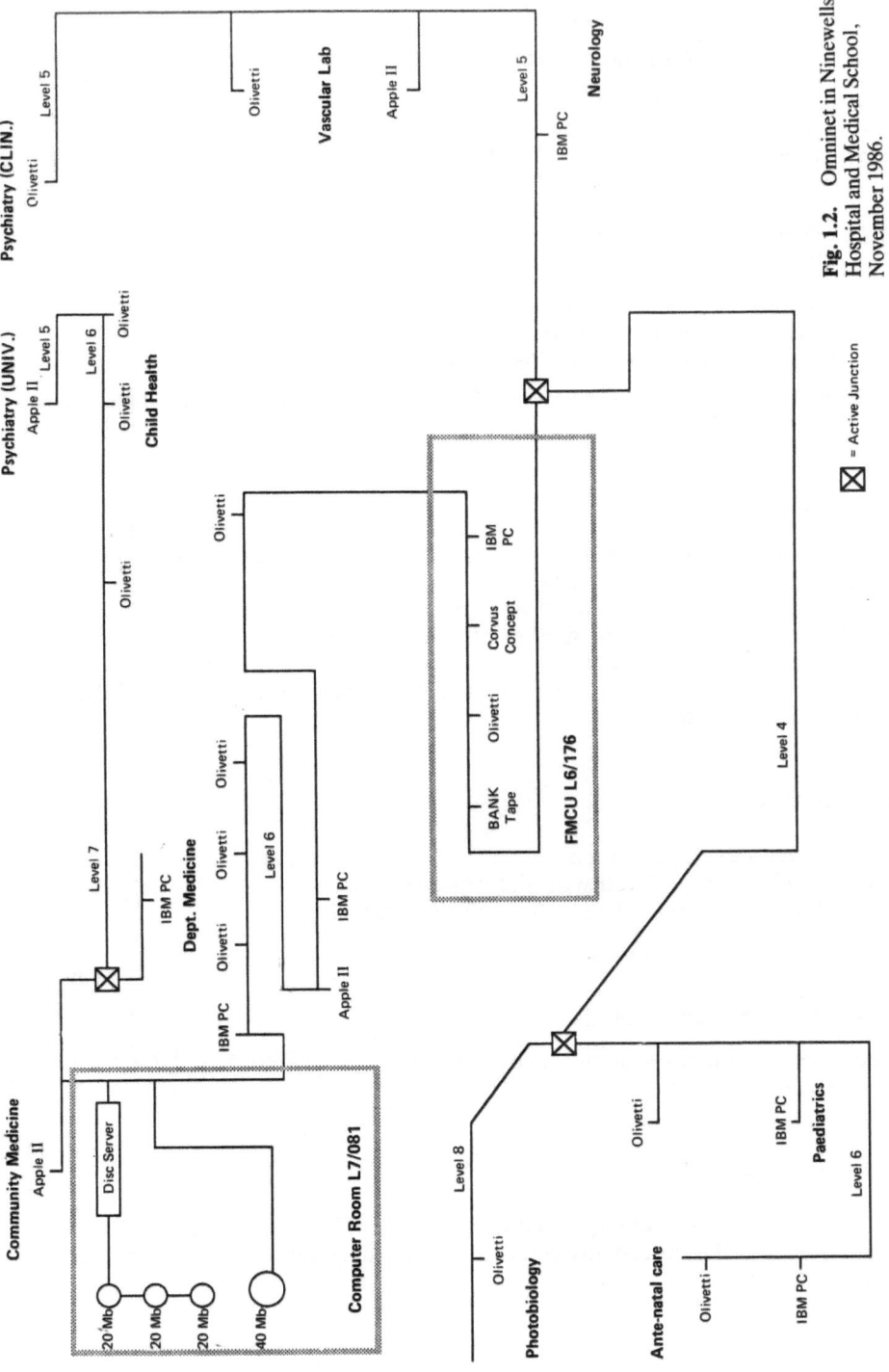

Fig. 1.2. Omninet in Ninewells Hospital and Medical School, November 1986.

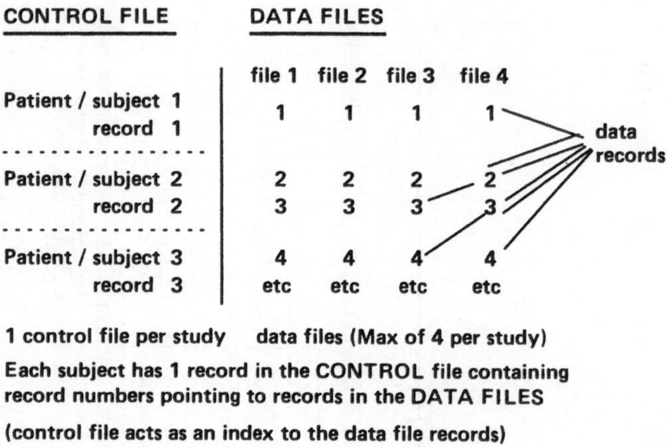

CONTROL FILE   **DATA FILES**

	file 1	file 2	file 3	file 4
Patient / subject 1				
record 1	1	1	1	1
Patient / subject 2				
record 2	2	2	2	2
	3	3	3	3
Patient / subject 3				
record 3	4	4	4	4
	etc	etc	etc	etc

data records

1 control file per study   data files (Max of 4 per study)

Each subject has 1 record in the CONTROL file containing
record numbers pointing to records in the DATA FILES

(control file acts as an index to the data file records)

Fig. 1.3. Craft file structure.

entry then acts as an index to all the data records relating to that subject within that application. A maximum of four datafiles may be generated for each study – each may contain over 100 fields of information in each record (Fig. 1.3). Data input and manipulation can take place across any or all of these files at any one time. The control file entry indexes all the data relating to an individual in chronologically ordered records so that information for instance on a patient may be held on the computer as in a formal medical case record. The control file may itself be indexed.

Program Suite

Craft has been developed in a modular fashion. This enables further modules to be developed and integrated with the present facilities as required. Up to now facilities have been divided into three distinct sections:

1. Generation of the database
2. Data input
3. Data manipulation, analysis and enquiry

The package is menu-driven, each facility being obtained through a series of step-down or step-up menus (Fig. 1.4).

Generating a Database

The user is free to define a database around his own application. Any information may be stored provided it can be accommodated by one of the following data types:

Dates
Integers

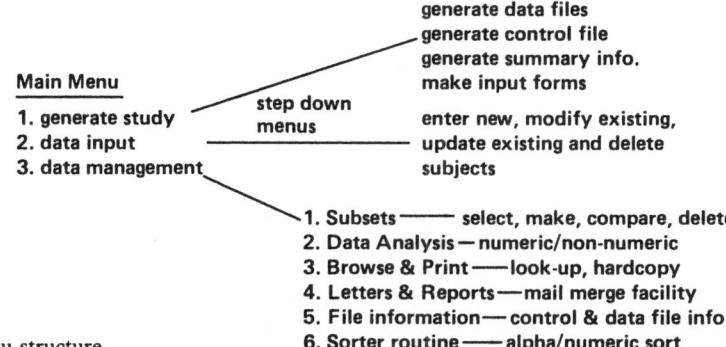

Fig. 1.4. Craft menu structure.

Reals

Free text

Single or multiple coded responses (chosen from a user defined dictionary)

Boolean (true/false)

These data types have been developed with medical data collection in mind and are therefore very supportive of non-numerical data. Certain of these data types, for example multiple coded response, are not available in other commercially available database systems. A multiple coded response is a field which enables the definition of a set of reply codes and associated expanded texts from which a number of codes can be input into that one field for example:

Question: What were the histological findings? *Reply*: [AC].

Possible answers: A, acute inflam; B, chronic inflam; C, granuloma; D, giant cells; E, paneth cells; F, transmural inflam.

The upper-case characters are described as "codes" while the associated texts are described as "expanded texts". In the example four different codes have been set as a maximum for input into this field.

Little knowledge of computing is required to set up a system, but careful planning and thought about the functions and expectations of the application and its database are essential. The Craft package allows the user to describe, on a simple question and answer basis, the data structures required by the particular application. A simple example is a file of patient registration records each of which is linked with further information about the same patient held in one or more "subsequent visit" files. The various control files that the package needs for "housekeeping" purposes are generated automatically. Each application may have up to four associated datafiles each with up to 100 fields. Multiple records can be entered and automatically linked, for each registered subject. This enables repeated information, for example periodic "follow-up" to be held and readily displayed and analysed. An important time-saving feature is the ability to stream the flow of input questions depending on the response to a "logical" type field. If, for example, the answer to the question "Does the patient have pain?" is "no" then all questions relating to the site, nature and severity of pain will be skipped.

Data Input

This includes all the facilities which allow the user to enrol new subjects, add information to existing subjects, modify previously entered information and, should the need arise, delete unwanted or redundant information. At all stages, validity checks are performed to ensure that the data being input fall within the limits defined by the user when generating the datafiles. Data input is speeded up by the creation of "input forms" which the user can define for frequent transactions such as entering review information. These ensure that only the questions relevant to a particular transaction are asked.

Database Management

The data manipulation and analysis facilities can operate across all the files. A number of mechanisms have been incorporated to enable the user to undertake various database enquiries.

Much of the power of Craft comes from the ability to create *subsets* or groups of subjects selected from the main database. Each of these subsets can be named and then saved to disc. Subsets can then be used to select patients for any of the Craft facilities for example selected mailings or further analysis and comparison with other subsets. Five types of subset can be created:

1. Time dependent, for example all patients who have had a third follow-up visit
2. Condition dependent, that is all individuals whose data satisfy a particular set of criteria, for example all males who have a Haemoglobin <10 with a positive biopsy finding
3. Dependent on comparing 2 numerical or date fields using the numerical operators ($<$, $>$, $>=$, $<=$, $=$) that is those with 5-year follow up or survival or with 12 months to diagnosis.
4. Sorted subsets; these are an extension of the other types. An ordered or *sorted* subset of patients can be created by sorting any of the alpha or numeric field types. These ranked subsets can then be used to produce reports, documents, letters etc in numerical or alphabetical order.
5. Manually entering the individuals to be entered into the subset.

A conditionally dependent subset may be defined with up to four conditions each of which may refer to a different file. Furthermore, once generated, subsets can be compared with other subsets creating a more refined subset.

Both *numerical* and *non-numerical analysis* facilities are incorporated as an integral part of the system. For the numerical data types, a suite of the more common statistical tests is provided (Fig. 1.5); however a large proportion of medical data is non-numerical but nonetheless needs to be studied. The two-dimensional table format is used to display this type of information (Fig. 1.6). Fig. 1.6 shows a two-way table comparing sex with site of disease; row and

A	:	Mean, Variance, STD, etc.
B	:	Regression Analysis Matched Pairs
C	:	T Test Unmatched Pairs
D	:	Wilcoxon Matched Pairs Signed-Ranks Test
E	:	Mann-Whitney Test
F	:	Mean, Mode, Median Percentiles, etc. Ungrouped Data
G	:	As (F) Grouped Data
H	:	Kendalls Test
N	:	No Stats Required

Fig. 1.5. Craft inbuilt statistical tests.   **Type Character**

column totals and percentage totals for each element are shown and the coding key is also displayed. Each analysis may be applied to all the patients or to any of the previously established subsets. The *browse* facility allows the user to choose specific data items. The system then "looks up" and steps through the records of any selected patient displaying each occurrence of the selected information. This is particularly useful when reviewing repeat visits in an out-patient clinic where rapid access and display of an individual's records is invaluable. *Letters* and *report documents* can be created from the information held in the database. This option can be used to generate recall letters, general practitioner bulletins, serial abstracts such as catalogues, summaries, address labels and other administrative material, again making use of the subset facilities where appropriate. In addition, standard letters can be prepared and saved for subsequent use with personalising information.

Several other utilities are available to aid in the operation of the system; these include a context-linked *help* facility which is indexed to the manual and data and subject file summaries.

System Requirements

The Craft system can be run on the IBM PC/XT/AT (and look alikes) and Apricot. A minimum configuration is 256 K RAM and two floppy disc drives although the use of a Winchester disc is strongly recommended.

Future Developments

The development of Craft's facilities is an on-going process. The numerical analysis section has recently been re-written while the subset facility is also being upgraded to increase the power of the subset facilities by providing the option to

Sex & Site of Disease
317 data points from a Sample of 317 subjects
Sample is from a population of 319 selected from ALL subjects

KEY for X axis
Field 36 in File crohns:cinv - EXTENT DISEASE
A = SMALL BOWEL
B = ILEO COLIC
C = LARGE BOWEL
D = DISCONTIN DISEASE

KEY for Y axis
Field 15 in File crohns:cgen - SEX
1 =   MALE
2 =   FEMALE

		?	A	B	C	D		TOTAL
	N!	0	0	0	0	1	!	1
?	%R!	0.0	0.0	0.0	0.0	100.0	!	
	%C!	0.0	0.0	0.0	0.0	2.3	!	0%T
	N!	5	46	35	26	16	!	128
1	%R!	3.9	35.9	27.3	20.3	12.5	!	
	%C!	45.5	47.4	37.2	36.6	36.4	!	40%T
	N!	6	51	59	45	27	!	188
2	%R!	3.2	27.1	31.4	23.9	14.4	!	
	%C!	54.5	52.6	62.8	63.4	61.4	!	59%T
	TOTAL!	11	97	94	71	44	!	317
	%T!	3.5	30.6	29.7	22.4	13.9		

N = number   %T = % of Total
% = empty fields   %C = Number as % of Column total
                              %R = Number as % of Row total

Fig. 1.6. Tabular data presentation and analysis.

have some of them dynamically updated as data are entered or modified. Greater power has been given to the mailmerge facility which enables formatted and smooth flowing letters and reports to be generated. The development of a graphics section is high on the list of priorities. The impending introduction of main-frame patient administration systems has also placed the development of a truly multi-user system and communication modules on Craft's critical pathway of development.

Applications Using the Craft System

Applications include the formation of disease registers, the collection of clinical data by units and patient administration systems.

Craft was piloted at an early stage in the development of a Crohn's disease register for Tayside region. This precursor system was set up to help in audit, research and patient management of the Crohn's disease population of Tayside. Clinicians seeing the facilities contained within this system felt that they too could utilise similar facilities within their own clinical practice. As it has developed, the range of studies to which it has been applied has steadily widened. At present 10 departments within the region of our own health board are using the system for one or more applications utilising the facilities to perform a variety of different functions. Most studies have been set up to perform a basic audit function, and many are also being used as a research tool. The recent increase in use of the package has resulted in the system gradually being introduced into areas relating to patient management. A waiting-list system has recently been introduced into the Urology Department and a General Practice system installed in a practice in mid-Wales. Currently the system is therefore used in the field of clinical audit, research and patient management.

Clinical Audit

The system is particularly valuable in this area as all data contained in a particular application can be audited in a number of different ways using the subset mechanism with the numerical and non-numerical analytical functions. Several disease registers have been generated including the initial Crohn's disease register and a register for bladder cancer. Both these applications are providing valuable types of audit information, for instance epidemiological – the incidence of Crohn's disease in the area has increased from 2.2 per 100 000 in 1968 to 4.9 in 1983. This type of information has also demonstrated the size of the bladder tumour problem within Tayside where 3420 cystoscopies have been performed on these patients over the past 16 years. Similarly the cost effectiveness of radiological investigation has been highlighted in the Crohn's disease study where it was found that the number of radiological investigations performed per patient on those known to have Crohn's disease has been increasing proportionately more than the increase in incidence and prevalence of the disease. Perhaps more importantly however the radiological audit has also shown that the proportion of normal results in this Crohn's population has increased dramatically over the past few years thus the rate of positive return for the standard barium meal and follow-through, barium enema and small bowel enema has decreased significantly. This it must be remembered is in the group known to have the disease and does not take into account those that have investigation for possible disease! Furthermore this type of audit has also demonstrated the inaccuracies of the Scottish in-patient morbidity statistics which showed that 530 individual patients had an in-patient ICD coding for Crohn's disease during the 16 years studied when in fact only 319 actually had the disease.

The package is also being used to audit deliveries in the obstetric departments of Tayside and will be used to produce the annual returns to the Health Board and the Scottish Office. Craft also operates in the Paediatric Department where similar information is collected as required by the Scottish Office on neonates and over the perinatal period – the SMR11 official data collection form. Facilities have been developed to transfer data to other computer systems and it would be possible to transfer this SMR11 information to the system in the Scottish Office either via modems or floppy disc. A similar local audit of the Special Care Baby Unit also uses the Craft system from which discharge letters are now printed routinely. For several years the psychiatric services in Tayside have logged patient contact data with a system based on the Health Authority's main-frame computer. Because of a number of factors, it has unfortunately proved to be extremely difficult for the clinician readily to retrieve information from that system and this fact, combined with the imminent demise of the software package on a change of operating system, has resulted in the psychiatrists choosing the Craft system to continue the data collection. One of the main reasons for this choice is the type of "hands on approach" which had been adopted to enable the clinicians to run analytical functions themselves. Three similar systems have therefore been created to manage each of the three health districts' psychiatric contacts.

Research Work

Many of the databases created for basic audit can also be used for further research on collected data. Interesting findings have already emerged from the Crohn's study where it has been found that the increase in frequency of Crohn's disease in elderly patients is mainly restricted to women who more often than not have been found to have large-bowel disease. Enquiry of the Bladder Cancer Register has shown that 5-year survival following cystectomy for bladder tumour is perhaps surprisingly high when it is considered that 90% of these operations are salvage cystectomies.

Several applications have been set up specifically as research projects including a gastric cancer trial sponsored by the Medical Research Council, a study into the effect of gut stimulant on ileus and a project investigating various parameters in normal and abnormal pregnancies. These are all on-going projects which will begin to produce their results in a few months' time. The Department of Neurology has begun a long-term study to monitor and investigate the epileptic population of the area.

Although many of these studies have been generated as research projects the databases created can also provide information on which to base further research. The technique of "going fishing" although not usually to be encouraged can be a useful adjunct in the routine audit systems and is only made possible by the rapid processing capability of the computer. We have for instance found that the frequency of Crohn's disease is particularly high in one post-code area, a small rural town. Initial enquiry revealed that this area had a different water supply and that the lead content was so high that measures to reduce it had to be taken because of European Economic Community regulations.

Patient Management

Several systems recently set up have moved into the area of patient management. This is however a different type of situation: the data are more dynamic in nature and speed of operation is an important consideration when the application is to be used daily by secretarial staff. This progression has resulted in further development of certain of the Craft facilities to enhance existing capabilities.

A urology waiting-list system has been created to oversee the waiting list and to perform basic monthly audits required by the health board. The system also generates lists of patients due for admission and letters telling patients when to come in to the hospital, and acts as a rapid look-up to see if an individual is on the list and indeed his position thereon. Ranked and ordered lists can be produced by age, date put on list, type of operation, consultant or indeed on any of the data contained within the system. This system is now being introduced into the management of the orthopaedic waiting list, with the possibility of many others following because of more detailed returns being required from 1988 onwards. A second and ambitious system has also been generated to help manage a large general practice in Wales. Many systems exist for use by general practitioners and all have advantages and disadvantages. This particular practice felt that the flexible and complex data manipulation facilities plus the potential for further development more than offset the risk of choosing a system whose origins were 400 miles from the practice and would make direct support a little difficult. The system itself contains an age/sex register, cardiovascular risk screening file, a diabetic recall monitoring section and well woman clinic which includes cervical smear data and recall, contraceptive data and breast examination information. It is hoped that this will be a precursor to further general practice orientated systems. Other proposed management systems which will shortly be created are an endoscopy system and a culposcopy and cervical cancer recall system.

Modular development of the system from a set of basic computing tools has enabled further modules to be created to perform specific tasks within a system with relative ease – of particular relevance in patient management systems. The gastric cancer register has a front end module which registers and randomises patients before entry into the study. The success of the neonatal audit resulted in a request for an intelligent discharge summary based on information contained within the system and has been introduced to the Paediatric Unit. The computerisation of diabetic clinics has long been at the forefront of computer utilisation in the medical field – we have therefore prepared a specific module to help in the monitoring of this group of patients in the diabetic clinic and have included data which will enable a shared care scheme to operate. Finally a module has been developed to enable the Craft system to be integrated with a commercially produced urodynamics system. This integration permits data produced within the urodynamic system to be transferred into the Craft database removing the need for manual input of information.

Although all the applications which have been discussed relate directly to the collection of medical data this need not be the case. We have at present one application which has been created as a reference bibliography. References are logged with the system which can then be searched by keywords, authors, journal, etc and then summaries or the abstracts from the paper printed out. Many other areas of potential application are in the pipeline.

Indeed though it is often difficult for a user to perceive the fact, his needs are often much more similar in basic structure to those of others than at first they might seem to him. This short summary has highlighted the versatility of this type of software approach. We however would be the first to agree it is *not* the answer to all clinicians' computerisation problems, but merely demonstrates one pathway a clinician may take and one possible approach to software development in the medical field.

Interfacing the Clinician and the Administrator

The Silicon Hospital

The silicon office has arrived. It might be defined as the interfacing of the relevant functions of each member of staff using an integrated information exchange system.

For many years now different aspects of hospital work have been computerised to a greater or lesser extent. These developments have in the main been confined to specific aspects of the service such as the diagnostic laboratories, radiotherapy treatment planning, other equipment-related systems and some medical record and administration functions. More recently immunisation and cervical cytology follow-up programs have evolved while at present much interest is being shown in computerised shared care schemes. The recording of morbidity returns – in Scotland the SMR series of documents – and some specific clinical data collection schemes have in the main been managed until recently by area computer departments. Unfortunately there has often been a widespread feeling that this has resulted in a one-way information flow with poor feedback to the clinicians.

Only since the development of the powerful microcomputer have clinicians become interested in clinically orientated data systems for audit, patient management and research. Using local microcomputers with software containing both patient management functions and facilities for direct analytical enquiry of the database clinicians have seen immediate and direct benefits from these clinical data systems. From the other direction developments in the areas of automating the management and administrative aspects of booking patients into hospital, assigning them to clinics, monitoring bed state and recording their discharge have evolved into the concept of Patient Administrative Systems (PAS).

There is however great potential for increasing the efficiency of both clinical and administrative systems if they could interact to their mutual advantage. For example the administrator and the clinician see the management of a waiting list through different eyes. The PAS will handle the mechanics of the task but the clinician takes this for granted and looks towards the computer to interact with him at unit or ward level and to provide audit and analysis of his medical practice. Similarly systems now emerging to enable shared care schemes to be implemented should be developed to enable them to exist in symbiosis with the PAS systems.

This feedback is the key to the clinicians' enthusiasm and hence determination to make a system work. It is the carrot which will encourage him to work with the administrator to achieve integration with the PAS systems.

With the cost of IBM PC compatible microcomputers now comparable with VDU terminals the adoption of such machines for user access to the PAS is being seriously considered for Tayside. The potential advantages of this type of PAS access are great. The diverse developments of specialist systems dedicated to specific areas including laboratories, radiology, nursing and even pharmacy present the challenge of offering direct access to these facilities which still rely heavily upon the transport of pieces of paper and the telephone. The interconnection of our laboratory system to our ward nursing system was well received by clinicians and by laboratory staff who were relieved of many telephone calls. A testimony of its value was the outcry when the facility was suspended. Other units have since been connected to our laboratory system gaining access through a mixture of microcomputers and terminals on minicomputers.

Is it possible to evolve an effective interconnected system which will integrate these different application systems into an effective information network? Some dedicated hospital systems, such as the laboratory system we support at Inverclyde Royal Hospital, already tap the facilities provided by a real-time PAS system for identification and matching of patients. It is now possible to make this type of connection through a hospital's own telephone network (DCX) using Data Over Voice (DOV) equipment. This DOV technique is already in operation in several hospitals although some have expressed reservations as to its ability to accommodate speech and the growing volume of data traffic on the comparatively narrow band width used by the system.

The microcomputer can now be armed with a repertoire of emulation software and a variety of connecting facilities. These range from simple RS232 VDU style connections to more sophisticated network connection protocols and enable the microcomputer to communicate with a number of different systems and then interact with the incoming data using its own processor.

It is quite likely that Tayside's new PAS will be based on ICL equipment which uses synchronous, page-orientated communication with its terminals. To implement a fully open network strategy to integrate it with the present and future systems this incompatibility will have to be overcome, for at present the hardware and software to connect one micro to a synchronous port can cost as much as the machine itself.

Perhaps the most powerful network medium is broad band with a capacity equivalent to thirty or more video channels – the technology from which it is derived. Indeed video images can be carried on the same medium as computer data. Computer-controlled video-image transfers are as yet largely an unknown quantity within health care practice but would be an invaluable medium for imparting information to patients, visitors and staff alike. The standard bulletin board facility could easily be extended to health education where interactive tele-video demonstrations or tutorials could be set up in clinics and waiting areas for use by patients, relatives and visitors. These facilities would also be valuable in the teaching of staff or students.

Is this all too fanciful and can we interface the diverse members of the team or teams better to cooperate in the provision of patient care, or is the prospect of the silicon hospital too daunting or indeed too threatening? Whatever our view the challenge is here.

Summary and Conclusions

The advent of the microcomputer suitable for use in the workplace has already made a significant impact on the provision of computing facilities in health care. The evolution of a multi-role software package has been traced from its origins to the wide variety of applications which it now supports with pointers to its potential further development.

The microcomputer has enabled data storage to be extended into clinical areas. When systems collect data as part of patient/clinic management functions with inbuilt data retrieval and analysis facilities it becomes possible to perform medical audit and research as valuable by-products, or perhaps some would see it as the other way round. Indeed this is at the heart of the notion of the two directions from which the benefits of computerisation are viewed, the administrator's and the clinician's.

With a speculative look to the future the prospects for integration of diverse medical computing systems have been explored by examining incremental and radical solutions. But the bringing together of the objectives of the clinician and the administrator will be the key if the greatest benefits are to come from the full introduction of new technology into health care. In this way both will see the advantages from administrative and medical audit giving accurate information upon which to base decisions for the short and longer term and from patient management which contributes to the quality of the provision of direct and shared care.

Perhaps the greatest hurdles come from the historical staffing structures within the Health Service. On the one hand there are so many diverse hierarchies responsible for different aspects such as records staff, clinicians, nurses, laboratory services etc and on the other there are computer departments steeped in main-frame experience. Many of the successful laboratory developments on minicomputers came from the lateral injection of staff and ideas, as are most of the microcomputer initiatives. But computer systems increasingly work across the traditional boundaries and will have a radical effect far beyond their immediate spheres of operation. How long will it take for all these diverse pathways of development to converge into the information systems which so many expect or even take for granted as being just around the corner? In other areas of computer applications outside the Health Service this future is already here. Will it come to us?

References

1 Carter NW (1971) Development of a computer system, based on a modular one, for pathology laboratories. IEE Conf Publ 79: 74–78

2 Carter NW, Griffith PD, White CJ, Chow MC, Lucas DF (1974) Design and implementation of a real time computer system for diagnostic medical laboratories. Medinfo 74: 975–978

3 Abson T, Prall A, Wooton ID (1977) Data processing in pathology laboratories: the Phoenix System 1. The overall design and the main facilities. Ann Clin Biochem 14: 307–314

4 UCSD p-system. Internal architecture (1981) Softec Microsystems Inc., San Diego, California

5 Netware product overview (1985) Novell Inc.

6 Walker MA, Bryce D, Carter NW (1986) A flexible clinical database. Br J Health Care Comput 3: 15–17

2 Incorporating a Microcomputer in the Surgical Office

D.C. Dunn

Introduction

With the introduction of new managerial concepts in the National Health Service clinicians are becoming more aware of the importance of keeping an audit. Having accurate and complete data available makes it easier to produce convincing arguments and to defend a budget. This is an area where computers should be of value but there are very few hospitals where a computerised system is used. This is largely due to a lack of software which is easy to use and to incorporate in the daily running of a surgical unit.

Over the last 6 years we have developed a system of surgical audit based on a microcomputer, and it is now in routine use in four consultant general surgical units in our hospital. In this chapter we will review our experience and describe the features of the system we have developed emphasising those which have enabled it to become part of our standard working practice.

In spite of the extravagant promises of the computer salesman the initial 3 years' experience showed that a computerised audit on its own was unlikely to survive as a long-term venture as the work involved in collecting the data was boring and an unacceptable addition to normal working practices. Data similar to those required for audit, however, were also being used to produce discharge summaries. This task was also tedious and in our hospital there was frequently a backlog of summaries for several weeks. We therefore concentrated on developing a method to improve the efficiency of production of discharge summaries and by this means supply the audit as a by-product. As a result we have been able to abolish the backlog of summaries and produce all the data we require. In response to the demands of our colleagues the present system is now being made available commercially.

This chapter describes the stages of development of the system and its use in practice, and tries to define some of the benefits found since its introduction.

History

The author has carried out some kind of audit on his firm for the last 13 years and this has been comprehensive, involving all in-patient admissions, since 1981. Initially the method used was manual and was based on recording all admissions in a pocket diary and analysing them at the end of each year. The diary method has the virtue of simplicity and as it will be used for comparison, it will be described briefly here.

Diary Method

It is the author's practice to give patients dates for proposed operations when they are seen in the out-patient clinic. Details are entered in a pocket diary. Emergencies and other extra admissions are then added to this diary at a weekly ward-round meeting. Columns are constructed for each day and simple one-letter codes are entered for each patient categorising the type of admission, grade of operation, the surgeon operating, complications and so forth. At the end of each month the numbers of codes in each column are added up and entered on a monthly chart. At the end of each year the monthly charts are combined to produce the annual statistics.

Computer Method

It was not long before computer experts began to suggest that the audit could be carried out much more simply and efficiently using a computer. As a result our initial computer system was purchased in 1982. This machine was a Superbrain QD microcomputer and used a database called Xcalibur which the author developed for surgical audit. Over the 3 years between 1982 and 1984 both the diary method and the microcomputer were used in parallel to record 3000 consecutive in-patient admissions. A comparison was made of the effort necessary to run an audit by both methods and the results were presented to the Association of Surgeons meeting in Birmingham in 1983.

Comparison of the Two Methods (see Table 2.1)

The diary method proved reliable and simple. The computer, when used for audit alone, proved very expensive and required four times the man hours for data input and verification even when time spent removing "gremlins" was excluded. However recall of data was much more efficient using the computer and individual cases could be rapidly extracted. Analysis by the diary method was useful though limited. This experience, the results of which may be surprising to those who believe computers can do everything faster and better than before, nevertheless convinced us that an audit carried out on a microcomputer had enormous potential. The extra time that it would require, however, would be a serious drawback.

Production of Discharge Summaries

We therefore turned to a study of the production of discharge summaries by the computer. The average time spent producing a discharge summary by the normal method of searching for data through the notes, dictating the summary and transcribing it was of the order of 15 minutes per patient. If the computer could produce an adequate discharge summary with 8 minutes' work, time could be saved and the production of the audit would become viable (Table 2.1).

Table 2.1. A comparison of the data collection times (for audit only) per patient using the diary or Superbrain with Xcalibur

Diary method	
Initial entry	1 minute
Weekly update	1 minute
	Total 2 minutes
(For 1000 patients/year: 33 hours per year or 40 minutes per week)	
Computer method	
Completing proforma	3 minutes
Verification and coding	1 minute
Entry to computer	4 minutes
	Total 8 minutes
(For 1000 patients/year: 133 hours per year or 2 hours per week)	

Important Principles

It became apparent that the whole exercise depended on strict control being kept over the amount of time to be devoted both to the collection of data and to its entry into the machine. A new computer system was therefore chosen and developed, keeping this principle in mind. The development relied both on our previous experience, and on continental trial and error in practice. The resulting package has proved acceptable both to the junior staff and to the medical secretaries.

In order to achieve this we found that:

1. The amount of data collected must be kept to a minimum. There was always a tendency to collect more data because of the ease with which it could be handled. It was quite easy for this to develop so that the computer system required more effort than the previous method of summary production.

2. Data entry must be facilitated by using as many techniques as possible to reduce the number of keystrokes required.

3. Coding decisions must be made easy and kept to a minimum.

4. Automatic validation by the software itself should be maximised thus reducing the chance of error.

5. Adaptability is essential in order to allow one to change the data that are collected and to carry out unpredicted analyses. If the program is not easily adaptable, more data will be collected because needs change from year to year. A non-adaptable program will have to be more widely based.

6. We also learnt that all the individuals who use the system have to feel some benefit from it personally. The secretary must find that her work is easier and less tedious. The junior staff must see that the production of discharge documents is easier using the system. We have found that the early clearance of notes from the juniors' desk provides the necessary inducement to keep the data collection going. Without these obvious advantages people tend to look for problems and the system fails or the staff leave.

The Present System

Hardware

We developed the system on a Sirius computer with a 10-megabyte internal Winchester disc. Back-up copies were made on 1 megabyte 5.25-inch floppy discs. We also had a Prism 80 Dot Matrix printer and an ACT Writer 30 daisy-wheel printer. The system will however run on many other microcomputers and is now available in a multi-user version of IBM compatible machines or the ICL Quattro, using Concurrent CPM or Concurrent PCDOS (Digital Research, California, USA).

Rescue Software

The program has been developed from a commercially available database package called Rescue (Grade One Computing Services Ltd). It also uses Wordstar (MicroPro International Corporation). The surgical audit package has been marketed as Dunnfile (Perthcrest, Perthcrest House, Cambridge Business Park, Milton Road, Cambridge CB4 4WT).

Rescue is a database program which can be freely adapted using an inbuilt menu-driven system without the need for knowledge of computer languages. Data are stored in fields which together contain 1024 bytes. The latter has proved ample for our purposes because of the ability of the program to store large amounts of data as single bytes (see below). The layout of the fields within a record is stored with a description and 19 different types of field are available, allowing storage of characters, numbers, dictionary entries, calculations from other fields and so on. A number of different descriptions can be applied to the same database allowing the production of different screen layouts and reports from the same data.

Records can be searched for using rules easily constructed by the user, and stored for future use. Selection rules are used to choose records with desired entries (e.g. all appendicectomies by one surgeon). More than 40 comparisons can be made in a single set of rules. Sort rules are used to print selected records in a defined order (e.g. by date of admission). Processing rules can be created which will alter the contents of selected fields within the database as defined by the user. The description and rules to use can then be incorporated in a menu option and used repeatedly if desired. Alternatively new rules can be made and used at any time by the keyboard operator. Within Dunnfile all these decisions about descriptions and rules have already been made and the system is ready for use.

Rescue also had several other features which attracted us.

1. It is possible to control entry of data thus ensuring accuracy. The program uses dictionary fields which will only accept entries chosen from a predetermined list and stored as a single byte. These dictionaries can either be short, using lists up to 29 characters in length, such as Emergency/Elective; or a full dictionary of up to 256 entries, each one up to 60 characters in length. Each of these 60 character entries is stored in the patient's record as their dictionary entry number, requiring only one byte of storage space. The entry can be made or recalled by typing in only enough letters to recognise it in the dictionary (e.g. APP will pick out appendicectomy). Wildcards can also be used (i.e. * representing any number of characters, or ? representing one character: e.g. *NDICE* will pick out appendicectomy).

2. Once the data are stored they can be manipulated by using alternative dictionaries which have different dictionary entries recalled by the same byte number. This can facilitate both data entry and analysis. Thus, the term "hernia strangulated" is easy to enter into a field (using HERN) but can appear in a letter as "strangulated hernia"; in the same way each operation can be represented by its ICD code, or operative BUPA grade, in an alternative dictionary. Also, as all entries are controlled by what is in the dictionary, the data are automatically validated.

3. The program can also link fields together so that unnecessary fields are not displayed at run time. Thus if there is no operation date the computer operator does not have to run through all the operative fields.

4. Rescue has a look-up facility so that data can be transferred from one database to another. Data therefore need only be entered once and then transferred automatically as required.

5. Word processing programs can be linked allowing reports to be generated using standard documents.

6. Data compression is possible. Apart from the data compression available by using dictionaries (1 byte represents 60 characters) Rescue also stores dates and numbers in a compressed form. Dates are entered very easily. The program will always enter the year last used unless prompted otherwise i.e. the date 19/10/1987 can be entered simply as 1910 (if the last date entered was also in 1987).

7. The inbuilt reliability was particularly impressive in comparison to other database programs we had tried. On three occasions, as a result of lightning strikes, the screen went blank while we were working on the databases. In none of these situations has it been necessary to re-copy the data from discs and no data apart from the record that was being worked on have been lost. Rescue has

a facility to bring the user back into the system at the point of any accidental exit and it then re-indexes all the files prior to normal shut down. This facility has meant that we have never lost data as a result of software failure. On one occasion the hard disc broke down and this is the only time we have had to restore from our floppy discs. With our previous Xcalibur program restoration from floppy discs was an almost weekly activity.

Organisation of Databases

The data are held in three main databases.

1. General practitioner details are entered in a GP Index. The majority of this information was entered when we started to use the system. Extra general practitioners are added as necessary.

2. Patient details are held in a second database called the Patient Index. Admission details which will allow us to run the waiting list and print the operating list are also entered into this part of the system. The details of each patient's general practitioner are brought across from the GP database automatically as the record is created.

3. In-patient details are held on the main database which also loads the relevant information about the patient from the Patient Index.

Using the System in Practice

Data Collection

Initial data on the patients and their general practitioners are collected in the out-patient clinic. At this time an addressograph label is stuck to a form and the patient's provisional diagnosis and proposed operation are recorded. Either at this time or at a later date the date of admission and date of operation may also be included on the same form. At the end of the clinic this form is handed to the computer operator who enters them into the GP database (if necessary) and the Patient Index. If patients are admitted off a waiting list their names, numbers, admission and operating dates are given to the operator when the admission is arranged.

When the patient is admitted to the ward a proforma is inserted into the notes. An addressograph is attached to this form by the ward clerk and the details required are filled in by various members of the medical staff as the patient goes through the hospital. The initial data such as admission date, and date admission arranged are entered when the patient is clerked by the houseman. Operative details can be entered by the surgeon and so forth. The proforma is completed at the time of patient discharge. If the fields have been filled in during the admission this final task takes only a few seconds.

When the patient attends for follow-up further data are collected. For all patients a note is made of number and name and they are graded from 1 (excellent) to 4 (bad) including a brief comment if necessary. The data for the first follow-up visit are added to the in-patient database and thus appear on analysis printouts.

Available Documentation

Instructions on how to use the system are kept available on the wards, in the secretarial office and in the operating theatres. These include details of how to fill in the forms and copies of the permitted dictionary entries.

Data Storage

The proforma is handed to the secretary who enters the details into the machine. While entering data on a patient the program automatically calculates the age, the total inpatient stay, the waiting time since the patient was seen in the clinic, and the postoperative stay.

One of the fields in the main database asks whether a discharge summary is required or not. If Yes is entered that record is selected when the discharge summary production facility is used. There is another facility which automatically changes this entry to No once the documents have been produced.

Documents Produced

There is no reason why the discharge document should not be produced on the day of discharge. We have not always been able to achieve this but we have reduced the delay in summary production from a few weeks down to a few days. Three copies of the document are made. The general practitioner's copy is made to be of such a size that it can be cut and folded into the standard GP note packet. The second copy is of a size which is compatible with the hospital notes and is filed there. The third copy is returned to the houseman. It contains the details which have been printed out but also several prompts. These suggest additional information which the houseman might send to the general practitioner. He can then dictate a relevant paragraph. This dictated paragraph can be added to a full discharge summary produced in the word processor by the machine. Initially about half of the patients were thought to require a full discharge summary in this way but this number has now dropped to less than 1 % with increasing expertise among the junior staff. They use the free-text fields on the proforma to insert enough information so that a full summary is unnecessary.

Once the documents have been produced the proforma is put aside for review by the consultant at the weekly ward round. The exercise of running through these proformas on a weekly basis has been found to be beneficial of itself in terms of patient care. Several outstanding problems are usually encountered and dealt with. At the same time the information on the computer is checked. If the information requires editing the proforma is returned to the secretary who makes the necessary changes on the database. The proforma can then be destroyed.

In addition to the discharge documents the prospective operating list for the firm is produced on a weekly basis by the machine from the data which have been inserted into the patient database. This is a simple report which is produced by Rescue without word processing.

Coding Method

In view of the need to keep the operating time to a minimum we rapidly discarded the use of complicated coding systems such as the ICD codes. The amount of time needed to look up an entry in the ICD coding book per patient would have caused the system to fail. We therefore developed a new system based on the use of the Rescue dictionary facilities. As far as operations and complications are concerned a simple dictionary was provided for each and the houseman encouraged to make a selection from it. As far as diagnoses were concerned three dictionaries were used. The first contained only the terms Right, Left or Bilateral. The second contained about 80 entries covering the names of various organs (e.g. hepatic, mammary, gastric etc). The third dictionary contained a list of about 90 conditions such as carcinoma, abscess, ischaemia etc. It was relatively simple for junior staff or secretaries to pick an entry from these lists and rapidly to become familiar with its use. It can be seen that a combination of the two main dictionaries gives an overall total of 7200 possible diagnoses. Thus a wide variety of possibilities could be covered without having to scrutinise huge lists of conditions.

Using the alternative dictionary facility it is possible to substitute all the entries in the operative dictionary by their ICD codes or BUPA grades. Operations can thus be graded automatically. It is also possible to use the combination of the two diagnostic dictionaries to produce an ICD code. Initially we felt no need to do this but the demands of others have led us to develop this facility. Even without it however the diagnosis we produce can be manually coded as previously and the standardisation and verification which the machine imposes improves the data which are available by this means.

Analyses

Analyses are usually carried out on a six monthly basis. It is also possible to use the machine to search for any individual patient, or group of patients, on an ad hoc basis. We have found this to be a great advantage, and searching for notes has become almost obsolete.

A very large volume of analyses can be produced from the computer but experience has shown that most of this is never used. Too much information is indigestible and as a result of our efforts of the last five years we have realised that only a few analyses are essential. These have been incorporated in the menu of Dunnfile. They include:

1. The number of admissions per consultant totalled per month and year
2. The number of admissions in certain diagnostic groups, such as gastric, oesophageal surgery, vascular surgery etc
3. The numbers of named operations performed over a period and the total
4. The numbers of each BUPA grade of operation performed

5. The details of all operations producing complications together with details of the complications
6. The operative experience and results of any one surgeon
7. The results of any named procedure including stays and complications

We rapidly found that analyses of simple complication rates, for example, were of little value. Having produced the figures we immediately wished to know why certain complications had occurred. A mortality rate of $N\%$ after aortic surgery was meaningless without information about the age of the patient, the diagnosis, and the cause of death. How many ruptured aortas were there for instance? And how many patients were aged over 80 years? We therefore print out a "mini" record of two or three lines per patient in such analyses, and this generally gives all the information required.

The Results of Using the System

Secretarial Training

Initially the system was run by a medical clerk with no secretarial or computer training. It took her about 2 weeks to learn to use it efficiently and there was no need to attend a formal course. More recently, trained medical secretaries have been able to pick up the technique in 1 or 2 days. We calculated that the total paid secretarial time required for the routine production of discharge summaries for the author, by the old method including administration, filing and breaks, was about 12 or 14 hours a week. Using the computer the secretary was able to produce the same volume of summaries working under 10 hours a week. The audit was produced as a bonus. There was thus a substantial saving in secretarial time.

Reactions of General Practitioners

We carried out a survey of the reactions of general practitioners to the format of the new summary. Fifty-one replies were received and 92% said that the communication produced by the computer had advantages over the usual discharge slip. They appreciated the extra information given. The particular format we produced was found to be acceptable by 83% and tolerable by a further 13%. Only two general practitioners did not like the document, commenting that it involved more reading than the previous handwritten discharge slip. When asked for individual comments the replies demonstrated that the majority liked having a document at the time of discharge containing most if not all of the essential details of the patient's admission. A legible document with an outline of the diagnosis, management and treatment was appreciated. Most of the other comments were about the size of paper which many felt should fit the "Lloyd George" notes or easily be folded into them. As a result of these comments we altered the size of the document and this produced further favourable reaction.

Other Benefits

Other benefits of running the audit included:-

1. Having an overview of the firm's activities which was not otherwise possible
2. Being armed with accurate figures for discussion
3. Being able to trace any patient with ease from one's own office
4. Being able to study and analyse complication rates

Recently the system underwent its biggest test when four new house surgeons started at a time when the program authors were away during a period of three weeks. The system continued to run without any problems and this demonstrates the ease with which it can be learnt, and the fact that staff left on their own prefer to work with the new system rather than the old.

Developments and Future Projects

One of the problems we have encountered is the delay before histology reports are available. This often means that the diagnosis cannot be entered initially in its final form. It may for instance be necessary to enter "breast lump" and to update this later to "breast carcinoma". To get over this difficulty we have developed a facility which sends a follow-up letter to the general practitioner when the histology is entered in the database. At the time of the production of this letter the diagnostic field can also be updated.

We have also developed the Patient Index so that the production of clinic letters is possible. This part of the system can also generate the waiting list in the computer and we are in the process of testing this facility in practice.

Rescue has been developed over the last two years so that it will run on the multi-user computer systems. This means that the secretary can run Wordstar and the various patient databases on the computer at the same time and more than one secretary can access the database at the same time. This has obvious advantages where several secretaries are working with data on the same machine. It is also possible to leave analyses running and get on with something else, such as word-processing letters.

Conclusions and Summary

Over the last 5 years the author has been interested in using a microcomputer for surgical audit. Comparison with a manual diary-based system showed that the time required to run a computerised audit alone would be prohibitive. A system was therefore designed to produce discharge summaries more rapidly than the routine method, and to produce the audit as a by-product. This system has been producing all the summaries for four consultant general surgical firms over the last 6 months and has proved acceptable and successful. Details of the system are given together with some of the results obtained.

Acknowledgements

The work on discharge summary development was done in collaboration with Mr R.F. Dale, Senior Registrar at Addenbrooke's Hospital, Cambridge, and his help has been invaluable. I am also grateful to our medical secretaries and numerous house staff who have patiently tried out various modifications.

3 Surgical Audit Using dBaseII

J.D. Holdsworth

Introduction

The purpose of this chapter is to give details of a computer program that was developed to store and audit information on surgical patients. Particular emphasis will be given to the way in which data were collected, the form in which they were stored and the presentation of subsequent analyses. Since there are many readily available publications covering the theory of computer programming the finer details of the programming involved will not be given, except where this clarifies the text.

A practising clinician will see and treat many patients with a variety of different diseases. To monitor these patients a record has to be kept of the numbers, the different diagnoses and treatments and the outcome of treatment. Such a breakdown or audit of clinical work, apart from being of importance for the individual clinician, has recently become increasingly important within the National Health Service where an emphasis has been placed on assessing clinical efficiency. Efficiency is most readily measured as patient turnover, either numbers per year or days in hospital, related to different diagnoses and treatments and, to some extent, can be determined from the data routinely collected in the records departments of most hospitals. However this form of data collection has a number of drawbacks. Coding of diagnoses and operations is not carried out by clinicians and there is no information available on the outcome of treatment, apart from a record of deaths. Thus there is a need for clinicians to collect their own data.

The collection, storage and audit of patient data is a continuing process. A single year's work will generate many thousands of items of information. Storage and later retrieval of such large amounts of information can only be carried out efficiently with the aid of computers. When he was appointed a consultant the author decided to keep records of his patients on computer from the time he commenced his duties. Although a few commercial computer software packages were available for this purpose they were found to be prohibitively expensive and therefore a decision was taken to develop suitable software from a relatively inexpensive programming language.

Aim

The main aim was to develop a computer program that would store and audit data on surgical patient admissions. A secondary aim was to make the program prepare discharge summaries so that patient data could be entered on computer by a consultant's secretary as part of her normal workload.

Choice of Software and Hardware

When making decisions concerning computer applications it is important to define the task to be completed by the computer, as above, and then choose software that will fulfil this requirement. Hardware should be selected to run the software.

To keep and store patient information a record subdivided into separate items of data, known as fields, has to be created for each patient. The term database is used to describe this process of keeping itemised records and can be applied equally well to information stored on conventional record cards or on computer. Thus the software requirement was for a package in which databases could be readily created and within which the data could be easily manipulated. Furthermore, to simplify data entry and reduce errors a high level programming language was also needed. The commercially available computer language dBaseII (Ashton Tate) was found to fulfil these requirements. An IBM personal computer with a 10 megabyte hard disc was chosen to run this software.

Development of Data Storage Software

Data Collected

In order to make data collection as accurate as possible and to avoid this process becoming a burden to both medical and secretarial staff it was considered important that the computer software developed to store patient records should not increase the amount of time normally spent preparing discharge summaries. The data collected were therefore limited to those items that would normally be used when compiling conventional discharge summaries. In order to standardise the information collected a form was developed (Fig. 3.1) to be completed by a member of the medical staff and from which a secretary could then transfer the data to the computer. Where additional text was to accompany a discharge summary this was dictated on a tape recorder and indicated, on the form, by ticking the appropriate box. The order in which information was placed on the form was governed by the order in which the computer was programmed to ask for each item. For those patients admitted to hospital for more than a day the whole form was completed, but for day-cases the information recorded on the form was limited to the first seven boxes, details of follow-up and either an investigation or an operation.

Structure of the Databases

Two databases were developed to hold the patient records (Fig. 3.2). One database was used to store the personal details of the patients (Names database), that is information that would remain the same for any subsequent admission when it would not need entering again. The second database (Admissions database) was used to store the clinical information generated by each admission. To link related entries in these two databases a single common field, unique to the patient concerned, had to be present in the records in each database. A patient's hospital number would normally have been suitable for this purpose. However, in Northumberland not all patients receive hospital numbers and therefore the computer was programmed to allocate a data number to each new patient record as it was created.

So that an audit could later be performed using only the Admissions database the patient's sex and admission number were recorded in this database as well as in the Names database. Also to assist with an audit the computer was programmed to calculate the age of each patient, from the date of birth, and place the result in the appropriate field in the Admissions database.

To reduce the number of items of information that had to be entered for each patient, software was developed to place code numbers for the consultant and hospital directly into each new record from system defaults, stored in the memory of the computer, which will be discussed later.

Dates were entered in the standard calendar format of day, month and year (DD/MM/YY). To simplify subsequent calculations on the dates of admission and discharge software was written to convert the calendar values of these two dates into the numeric Julian [1] equivalents. The numeric form was then stored in the appropriate fields in the Admissions database. The number of days in hospital was calculated, by the computer, as the difference between the dates of discharge and admission plus one day to avoid patients admitted and discharged on the same day from being in hospital for zero days.

Two additional databases were created to hold the codes needed for the information stored in the patient databases. One of these databases was designed to hold a code number, the name and address for each of the local general practitioners (GP database). This database also stored the names of all the consultant clinicians working within the hospital group and for whom additional copies of discharge summaries were sometimes required (Fig. 3.1, box 3). The second additional database was designed to hold the International Codes [2,3] (Codes database) for diagnoses and operations. Previous medical history and complications were also selected from the diagnoses stored in this

1. PATIENT DETAILS

       Surname
       First name
       Address
       Hospital number
       Date of birth
       Sex

       GP

2. ADMISSION TYPE

      1. Daycase   ( )
      2. Waiting list   ( )
      3. Emergency - GP/Casualty   ( )
      4. Emergency - Internal   ( )
      5. Internal referral   ( )
      6. Direct from GP   ( )

3. EXTRA COPIES OF SUMMARIES   Yes ( ) No ( )

      How many extra copies?   ( )

      For whom?

4. DATES

      Admitted
      Discharged/died

5. DIED, INTEREST

      Died   Yes ( ) No ( )

      Interest   Yes ( ) No ( )

6. DIAGNOSIS (base on histology, include side of body)

      Principal

                     Left/Right

      Secondary

                     Left/Right

7. Is this admission a complication of treatment during
a previous admission?
                     Yes ( ) No ( )

8. PAST MEDICAL HISTORY   Yes ( ) No ( )

      1.

      2.

      3.

      4.

9. INVESTIGATIONS   Yes ( ) No ( )

      1.

      2.

      3.

---

10. TREATMENT

      1. Surgical   ( )
      2. Medical   ( )
      3. None   ( )

      Details of treatment (ie operation)

      1.

      2.

      Date   Grade of surgeon ( )

11. COMPLICATIONS (up to 3)   Yes ( ) No ( )

      Wound   Infection   ( )
                Dehiscence   ( )
                Haematoma (bruising)   ( )
                Haemorrhage (bleeding)   ( )
                Necrosis skin edges   ( )

      GI   Paralytic ileus   ( )
                Anastomotic leak   ( )
                Jaundice   ( )
                Cholangitis   ( )
                Subphrenic abscess   ( )
                Pelvic abscess   ( )
                Pancreatitis   ( )
                GI bleed   ( )

      Respiratory   Chest infection   ( )
                Pneumothorax   ( )
                Respiratory failure   ( )

      CVS   Arrhythmia   ( )
                MI   ( )
                Cardiac failure   ( )
                DVT   ( )
                PE   ( )
                CVA (stroke)   ( )
                Limb ischaemia   ( )

      Urinary   Retention urine   ( )
                UTI   ( )
                Renal failure   ( )

      Miscellaneous Clotting disorder   ( )
                Allergy   ( )
                Side effect drug   ( )

      Other (enter details)

12. SECOND OPERATIONS   Yes ( ) No ( )

      1.

         Date   Grade of surgeon ( )

      2.

         Date   Grade of surgeon ( )

13. FOLLOW UP

      Where?   Ashington ( )   On ward   ( )
             Morpeth   ( )   Readmission   ( )
             Alnwick   ( )   Entered on WL   ( )
             Berwick   ( )   To be arranged ( )
             Blyth   ( )   None   ( )

      When?   Weeks   ( )

---

14. TEXT Yes ( ) No ( )

Field names	Field size (bytes)	Storage format	Comment

NAMES DATABASE (personal details of patients)

1. Data number‡	6	Number	Allocated to each patient at initial entry in database
2. Name	30	Text	Entered as surname followed by first name (eg Smith, John)
3. Address	50	Text	
4. Hospital number	8	Number	
5. Date of birth	8	DD/MM/YY	
6. Sex‡	1	M/F	
7. General practitioner	3	Code number	Extracted from a database containing all the local GPs and their addresses
8. Admission number‡	2	Number	Incremented by 1 for each readmission

---

ADMISSIONS DATABASE (clinical details of admission)

1. Data number‡	6	Number	
2. Age	2	Number	Calculated from date of birth as above
3. Sex‡	1	M/F	
4. Admission number‡	2	Number	
5. Consultant	1	Coded	
6. Hospital	1	Coded	
7. Type of admission	1	Coded	Daycase, waiting list, emergency, etc
8. Date admitted	5	Number	Julian date calculated from date entered as DD/MM/YY
9. Date discharged or died	5	Number	As for date admitted
10. Days in hospital	2	Number	Calculated from dates admitted and discharged + 1 day
11. Died	1	Y/N	ie yes or no
12. Interest	1	Y/N	
13. Diagnosis	14	Coded+	Up to 2 + side of body
14. Previous medical history	24	Coded+	Up to 4
15. Investigations	18	Coded+	Up to 3
16. Management	1	Coded	Surgical/medical/none
17. First operation	21	Coded+	Up to 2 during one anaesthetic + date (DD/MM/YY) & grade of surgeon as a number
18. Second operations	30	Coded+	As first operation, but since this can be 2 separate operations 2 dates and 2 surgeons can be entered
19. Complications	24	Coded+	Up to 3 + if subsequently re-admitted with a complication the diagnosis of the second admission placed here
20. Follow up	3	Coded	A combination of the place for followup and the time to followup (see figure 3.1)
21. Text	940	Text	Not stored

---

‡ Information duplicated in the 2 databases.
+ 6 figure code numbers extracted from Codes database containing diagnoses, treatments and investigations.

Fig. 3.2. Details of patient databases.

database. Investigations, excluding routine blood tests, were allocated codes and also stored in the Codes database. Each record in the Codes database was subdivided into three fields. One field stored the International Code and a second field a descriptive title to accompany this code. The third field in each

---

⬅

Fig. 3.1. Form used for patient data collection.

record was for a search code used to assist in the location of the correct information from within this database. These search codes are discussed in detail below. When entering a patient record, once the correct diagnosis, operation or investigation was located in the Codes database, the International Code was placed in the relevant field in the Admissions database and the descriptive title printed on the discharge summary. Similarly once the name of the correct general practitioner was located in the GP database the code for the general practitioner was placed in the GP field in the Names database and the name and address placed on the summary.

In certain areas these International Codes were found to be limiting. For example, the majority of vascular bypass operations were covered by a single code number. Where such a limitation was encountered further additional codes were created by adding a letter as a suffix to the nearest appropriate International Code. Within the Codes database all International Codes were prefixed by a letter to distinguish between diagnoses, operations and investigations. The maximum size of a code number was 6 characters (bytes) and codes were therefore stored in blocks of 6 characters in the Admissions database. Currently there are 984 records in the Codes database, 604 diagnoses, 328 operations and 52 investigations.

Some fields in the patient Admissions database had additional information stored with the International Codes. For example, the side of the body, where appropriate, was stored with the diagnoses and operations also included the date on which they were performed and the grade of the operating surgeons.

Program Files

The program was developed as a number of modules each containing a suite of computer files designed to operate the functions of that module. One module dealt with the patient records. A second module performed the audit on these records and a third module allowed new codes to be entered into the Codes and GP databases. This third module also printed alphabetical lists of diagnoses, operations and investigations to assist with the preparation of discharge summaries. The program was written so that all input from the computer keyboard was in response to questions displayed on the screen. Thus any person using the program could do so without prior knowledge of programming in dBaseII.

When the computer was switched on the system booted from the hard disc and in so doing asked for the date and a password before access to the program was permitted. The date was subsequently printed on the discharge summaries and the password routine was developed to protect the data stored on the hard disc. Providing that the correct password was entered an introductory message was displayed on the screen to indicate that control of the computer had been handed to the patient program. This message was followed by a menu from which one of the three modules, described above, was selected. The module designed to get patient data also contained a facility which allowed the records of patients already stored on the computer to be retrieved and, if necessary, modified. Entry of each new patient record was preceded by a menu from which the computer operator could choose to enter patient data. The other alternatives available from this menu were to change the system defaults or to print the discharge summaries. When this menu was on display the system defaults were also shown in one corner of the computer screen. The system defaults consisted of information which was stored by the computer between sessions and which only needed changing occasionally to suit individual patient entries. These defaults were; the name of the consultant for whom the discharge summaries were being prepared, the name of the hospital to which the patient was admitted, the initials of the persons collecting and entering the data, and the number of copies of each summary to be printed routinely. The consultant and hospital were selected from lists of those available to the system.

Data entry followed the order listed in Fig. 3.1 and, with the exception of the personal details and the dates of admission and discharge, was from menu selections. The surname and hospital number were entered first. The computer than checked to see if the patient had been admitted before. If there was a previous record in the computer all the personal details of that patient were displayed for checking, whereas if there was no previous entry the operator was prompted, by the computer, to enter the personal details. All keyboard entries were displayed after completion so they could be checked and error trapping was performed, by the computer, so that unacceptable key strokes were rejected. Should there have been a previous admission then the computer operator was asked whether or not the current admission resulted from a complication of the treatment given previously (Fig. 3.1, box 7). If this was the case then the diagnostic code entered for the current admission was also placed by the computer in the complications field of the last admission. As a final entry for each patient up to 14 lines of text (940 characters) could be entered. Once completed the record for that patient could be re-displayed and, if necessary, altered. The computer was now ready to accept data for another patient and indicated this by re-displaying the menu from which a data entry had commenced.

International Codes were found from within the Codes database using the search codes. A search code consisted of up to four letters and since indexing of databases speeded up data retrieval, the Codes database was indexed on this field. The first letter of a search code denoted the data type (diagnosis, operation or investigation), the next two letters identified the appropriate site in the body and the fourth letter, used with diagnostic codes only, denoted pathological disease groups. To search for information from this database the correct search code had to be compiled in the memory of the computer. The computer was programmed to allocate the first letter to the memory, but the next three letters were allocated by input from the keyboard in response to three menus (Fig. 3.3) which appeared sequentially on the screen. The first menu was based on the systems of the body, but included some additional subjects that did not conform to the system groups. The content of the second menu varied according to the choice made from the first menu and was a list of organs or tissues found within the system selected. The third menu, used only when searching for a diagnosis, was a list of pathological disease groups. Investigations were located using a modification of the first menu only. Once a search code was compiled in the computer memory this code was compared with the search codes stored in the Codes database and for all occurrences of a match between the two codes the computer displayed on the screen the descriptive title accompanying each International Code. The final choice of the correct descriptive title was then made by the computer operator from those on display. Thus, with reference to

```
FIRST MENU                        SECOND MENU                    THIRD MENU
(Systems of the body with         (Organs within the system      (Diagnostic groups)
some additional options)          selected. This example for
                                  gastro-intestinal system)
-----------------------------------------------------------------------------------------
A)  BLOOD AND LYMPHATICS          MOUTH AND THROAT               ARTERIAL DISEASE
B)  CARDIO-VASCULAR               OESOPHAGUS                     CONGENITAL
C)  GENITO-URINARY                STOMACH                        DEGENERATIVE/AGING
D)  GASTRO-INTESTINAL             DUODENUM                       INFECTION/INFLAMMATORY
E)  GLANDS (endocrine and exocrine) SMALL BOWEL                  ISCHAEMIA/INFARCTION
F)  HEPATO-BILIARY                APPENDIX                       OBSTRUCTION
G)  HERNIA                        LARGE BOWEL                    OVERACTIVE (hypertrophy)
H)  MUSCULO-SKELETAL              ANUS/PERINEUM                  TRAUMA (injury)
I)  NERVOUS                       ABDOMEN (not classified)       TUMOUR (benign & malignant)
J)  RESPIRATORY                   GENERALISED DISEASE            UNDERACTIVE (failure/atrophy)
K)  SKIN                          SYMPTOM                        PREVIOUS TREATMENT OR OPERATION
O)  ANATOMICAL NAME                                              NOT CLASSIFIED
M)  INFECTIOUS DISEASE
N)  COMPLICATION
O)  METABOLIC
P)  NOT CLASSIFIED
-----------------------------------------------------------------------------------------
```

Fig. 3.3. Details of menus used to search for diagnoses and operations.

Fig. 3.3, in order to find a diagnosis, for example carcinoma of the sigmoid colon, the computer would allocate the first letter (D) and entry of D, G and I from the keyboard as each search menu was displayed would create the search code DDGI. All colonic tumours were indexed on this search code and would therefore be displayed on the screen.

```
                          Northumberland Health Authority
ASHINGTON HOSPITAL
West View
Ashington
Northumberland   NE63 0SA

Telephone :Ashington 812541
----------------------------------------------------------------------------------
CV/JH                                                                     04/04/86

     Dr P White
     The Health Centre
     MORPETH

PATIENT                : Holdsworth, John (Dob 02/02/50; Unit no 023456)
                         25 Stream Avenue, Morpeth

ADMITTED               : 01/03/86

DISCHARGED             : 10/03/86

TYPE OF ADMISSION      : Elective

DIAGNOSIS              : Inguinal hernia (Left)

INVESTIGATIONS         : Gastroscopy
                         Ba enema

OPERATION              : Repair inguinal hernia

COMPLICATIONS          : Bronchopneumonia
                         Wound infection

SUMMARY                : Admitted for treatment as indicated.  Known to suffer
                         from chronic obstructive airways disease.
Post-operative recovery complicated by a severe chest infection and a low
grade wound infection both of which had improved by the time he was
discharged.

FOLLOW UP              : Morpeth Cottage Hospital, 6 weeks


JD Holdsworth, MD FRCS
Consultant Surgeon

cc Dr J Smith
   Ashington Hospital
```

Fig. 3.4. Example of a discharge summary.

Discharge Summaries

The layout of the discharge summaries is illustrated in Fig. 3.4. Where there were no data for a particular line of the summary that line was omitted. To economise on the amount of data stored on the hard disc the text accompanying each discharge summary was deleted once it had been printed. For routine uncomplicated operations additional text was often not required since all the information needed was printed within the headings of the summary.

Development of the Audit Software

Audit was developed for either a single year (annual audit) or for a group of patients selected by entries from the keyboard (user-defined audit). The annual audit was broken down into broad diagnostic groups (e.g. deaths, emergencies, upper gastro-intestinal tract, vascular), whereas the user-defined audit was developed so that a group of patients could be selected for analysis on up to eight of the fields available in the Admissions database (Fig. 3.5). A number of routines were developed to count those patients selected for analysis. Examples of the output from some of these routines are given in Fig. 3.5. The first table illustrates the output from an initial count. To maximise the information available from this count all possible data pairings were counted and then tabulated in the form of a triangular grid from which the result obtained from any pair of variables could be found. To clarify the table all zero pairings were omitted. The next three tables (Fig. 3.5) present diagnostic and operative information for the same group of patients. The data on the second and third tables were placed in descending order of frequency of diagnosis and operation respectively and were on similar fields to those used by the initial count. The fourth table gave additional information concerning the operations so that those diagnoses and complications associated with each operation could be identified.

Capability Program

The program files used by the three modules occupied 0.60 megabytes of disc space, with a further 0.19 megabytes being used by the GP and Codes databases. During the year 1985 there were 1592 patient admissions and storage of data from these patients occupied a further 0.62 megabytes of disc space. Thus, in its present form, the program will run for more than 10 years before the capacity of the hard disc is exceeded.

Conclusions and Future Developments

The program has been running since October 1984 with an annual audit prepared for 1985. During this time it has undergone a number of modifications, but has remained in its present form for the last 9 months. During the first year considerable effort was required to develop the software so that it was suitable

1. INITIAL COUNT

	Total	Secop	Died	Comp	NoRx	Med	Opn	Int	EmInt	EmErt	Elect	Dayca	DayHo	Age	Women	Men	Ad>1
Totals	30	6	5	12			30			18	12		37	72	10	20	12
Admission>1	12	2	2	5			11			5	7		33	71	3	9	
Men	20	5	3	9			20			13	7		34	71			
Women	8	1	2	2			10			5	5		40	73			
Mean age	72	69	79	74			72			72	72						
Days hospital	37	51	36	42			37			41	32						
Daycase	.																
Elective	12	1	3	5			12										
Emerg External	18	5	2	7			18										
Emerg Internal																	
Internal ref																	
Operations	30	6	5	12													
Medical treat																	
No treatment																	
Complications	12	6	5														
Died	5	1															
Second opn	6																

2. DIAGNOSTIC COUNT

Diagnosis	Total	Adm>1	Men	Women	Age	DayHo	Dayca	Elect	EmErt	EmInt	Int	Opn	Died	Comp
1 Rest pain leg	11	6	7	4	72	31		7	4			11	2	4
2 Gangrene foot	7	3	5	2	74	32		2	5			7	1	3
3 Gangrene leg	8	3	4	4	66	55		3	5			8	2	4
4 Iliac occlusion	2		2		68	43			2			2		
5 Superficial femoral occlusion	1		1		78	58			1			1		1
6 Trauma to leg	1		1		45	16			1			1		

3. OPERATIVE COUNT

Operation	Total	Men	Women	Age	Dayca	Elect	EmErt	EmInt	Int	Cons	SR	Reg	SHO	HO	Died	Comp
1 Below knee amputation	24	16	8	72		12	12			15		9			4	11
2 Above knee amputation	6	4	2	70		6				3		3			1	1

4. OPERATION, DIAGNOSIS AND COMPLICATIONS COUNT

Operation	Total	Diagnosis	Total	Complications	Total
1 Below knee amputation	24	Rest pain leg	11	Wound infection	6
		Gangrene foot	7	Wound dehiscence	2
		Gangrene leg	5	Cardiac arrest	2
		Superficial femoral occlusion	1	Cerebro-vascular accident	2
				Acute retention urine	2
				Bronchopneumonia	1
2 Above knee amputation	6	Gangrene leg	3	MI	1
		Iliac occlusion	2	Wound infection	1
		Trauma leg	1		

Fig. 3.5. Example of the tables produced by an audit of amputations.

for use by a secretary. Once the program was ready a secretary was taught to use the computer in a single session. The only input now required to the program, by the author, is to remove minor programming errors, as they are identified, and to enter new International Codes. Data entry has been found to be acceptable to the secretarial staff who have expressed a preference for using the computer to prepare discharge summaries, since there are fewer typing errors and when errors do occur they can be corrected more readily than on a conventional typewriter. Preparing summaries on the computer has not increased the amount of time normally devoted to this task. The program has therefore achieved the objectives outlined earlier.

The main limitation of the present version of the program results from the inability of dBaseII to deal with the entry of large blocks of data, such as text, which may be of variable length. It is for this reason that the text entries are destroyed after printing since each entry led to the full 940 characters being stored irrespective of the length of the entry. As a result the complete version of a discharge summary cannot later be retrieved from the computer. To store this text permanently would lead to the capacity of the hard disc being exceeded within 3–4 years. This limitation could be overcome if the computer language provided for fields of variable length which only occupied disc space relative to the amount of information entered. The manufacturers of dBaseII have recently addressed this problem with an improved computer language, dBaseIII (Ashton Tate), which has fields of variable length. Unfortunately this variable field can only be used by a computer operator who has a working knowledge of programming in dBaseIII and therefore, in its present form, this field is not suitable for the software application illustrated in this article in which there was a requirement for the computer to be operated by a person lacking programming expertise. If future versions of dBaseIII address this difficulty then the present program will be converted to dBaseIII so that text can be stored as well as the coded information. A further development would be to write software to store information on surgical out-patients who would generate large volumes of text, in the form of letters, in addition to some coded information. Since the majority of patients are listed for surgery following a visit to the out-patient clinic a logical extension of such a development would be to operate the surgical waiting list from the computer.

References

1 Castro L, Hanson J, Rettig T (1985) Advanced programmers guide. Ashton Tate, Culver City
2 International classification of diseases (1978) World Health Organisation, Geneva
3 Classification of surgical operations (1975) Office of Population and Censuses and Surveys, St Catherines House, London

4 The Development of an Operation Mortality Index on Microcomputers

S.J. Nixon

Introduction

Many health service reports have advocated the development of clinical care evaluation. These include the Cogwheel reports, the Brotherston report in Scotland and the Royal Commissions on Medical Education and the National Health Service. Despite these recommendations little real progress has been made either at a local or at a national level.

In the field of audit, surgeons are in a favourable situation compared with many of their professional colleagues in that they are able accurately to describe and quantify their work. Internationally accepted codes of disease and operations exist and well-established criteria of success and failure are also available. Death within thirty days of surgery represents the most reliable indication of failure and the need for careful consideration of avoidable factors.

The collection of in-patient hospital statistics is a statutory obligation of National Health Service hospitals and, ideally, audit should be a by-product of this routine, administrative work. However these data have been subject to serious criticism regarding their accuracy and completeness. Excessive delay in production further erodes their relevance to the clinician. The main reason for inaccuracy is the multiple steps in data transfer from a clinical action to computerisation and analysis. There are many specific factors which contribute to the poor performance of hospital systems for data capture. These include lack of interest by doctors and insufficient knowledge of discharge details to code for data collection. It is unlikely that there will be sufficient improvement in the near future to make hospital data of real clinical value.

History of Lothian Surgical Audit

Audit in Lothian (Edinburgh) originated at the time of Lister but the present-day system was instigated by Sir James Learmonth who, in 1946, established the principle that any death following surgery should be discussed amongst colleagues in a constructively critical manner. Since that time surgeons in Lothian have voluntarily collected statistics of their in-patient and out-patient work together with details of each patient who died whilst under surgical care. These data are presented to surgical colleagues for critical comment, a form of peer review. In 1979 a sub-committee of the Division of Surgery was set up to attempt to coordinate this data collection so that annual reports might be produced including an analysis of the 15 surgical teams in the 8 hospitals of the Lothian Area. All general, vascular and urological surgeons in the Area agreed to participate.

Between 1979 and 1982 the task of collection and analysis of the data (25 000 operations and over 400 deaths annually) was undertaken at a central office. A system was developed in which a tear-off slip was detached from each operation report. This stated the pathological process and operation type. These slips were collected at the audit office for filing and manual analysis. During this period there was regular discussion between surgeons and community medicine specialists. It soon became apparent that internationally accepted codes of disease and operations were inadequate for audit purposes. A unique coding system was therefore developed which had considerable audit potential. Between 1979 and 1982 annual reports were produced including the operative mortality details and commentaries from nominated consultants who were asked to discuss those areas of surgery where performance might be criticised. Individual surgeons were encouraged to compare their own performance with that of their colleagues combined. The audit data became a focus for discussion between surgeons and this lead to changes in practice.

Despite the relatively small data set collected from each patient, the manual system was expensive to operate both financially and in time. The research grant was terminated in 1982 and a low-cost alternative to the manual data handling was urgently required if the advantages of the previous 4 years were to be maintained. The audit committee obtained a grant in order to employ a full-time secretary for one year. A Cromemco 64K RAM microcomputer was made available. The requirements of the system were precisely understood. The coding system which had been developed divided the operative procedures into 16 broad areas of anatomy. Each area was subdivided into pathologies and each operation type was also coded. As a result, an operation with its pathological indication could be precisely defined by three code numbers, each up to two characters in length. It was necessary to have the facility to store information on 25 000 operations. The patient was to be identified by his/her unique hospital number (up to 10 characters). Emergency procedures, known to have a high morbidity and mortality, were flagged.

At this stage the intention was to analyse the operation workload for each surgical team annually and to combine the data from all units into an Area Report. No sort or search facilities were required. The programs were written in BASIC by medical staff and introduced in 1982 in two units with experience in microcomputing. In the remaining units the data were analysed manually.

During this year the computer system proved to be successful and was used to analyse the complete data for 1983. The operation/mortality analysis for 1983 was produced within 3 months and the completed annual report in 6 months. The value of the microcomputer was clearly demonstrated and its place established.

During this introductory year, when surgeons were more actively involved in coding and computing, many lessons were learned. The Cromemco microcomputer, now 5 years old, was proving to be unreliable and expensive to maintain. The coding system, although based on 4 years of study, was still deficient in a number of key areas. The remoteness of the central office from the surgeons themselves was an obvious handicap when compared with the two units who were actively involved in data handling. It was considered essential to return the responsibility for the completeness and accuracy of the data to the individual surgical units. The microcomputer system was able to handle a larger data set and thereby offer many additional facilities to the surgeons. In response to these realisations the present audit system was designed and developed.

The Lothian Surgical Audit Computer System

Overall Aim

The Lothian Audit system remains entirely voluntary. Our aim is to collect high-quality data about the operations performed in our Area and the diseases for which these procedures are done. We collect data from all general, vascular and urological surgeons in the Area and have recently included the oral surgeons and data from a team of surgeons from a neighbouring Area. This information is pooled to allow calculation of the operation and disease mortalities. The tables produced are published annually together with a critical analysis of our performance as a group. We return to each surgical team an analysis of their collective experience allowing a comparison with the Area results. More recently we have been able to give individual consultants an analysis of patients under their care and to individual surgeons an analysis of patients on whom they have operated.

Technique of Data Acquisition

Operation Statistics

On completion of an operative procedure the surgeon dictates an operation report. This report is typed and contains a standard header which specifies the data required for the audit system. Ideally, at the time of dictation or soon after, the surgeon codes the procedure using our codes. After typing the operation summary, the secretary removes the tear-off slip from the report and it is kept either in the unit for input to the computer or sent to the central office (Fig. 4.1).

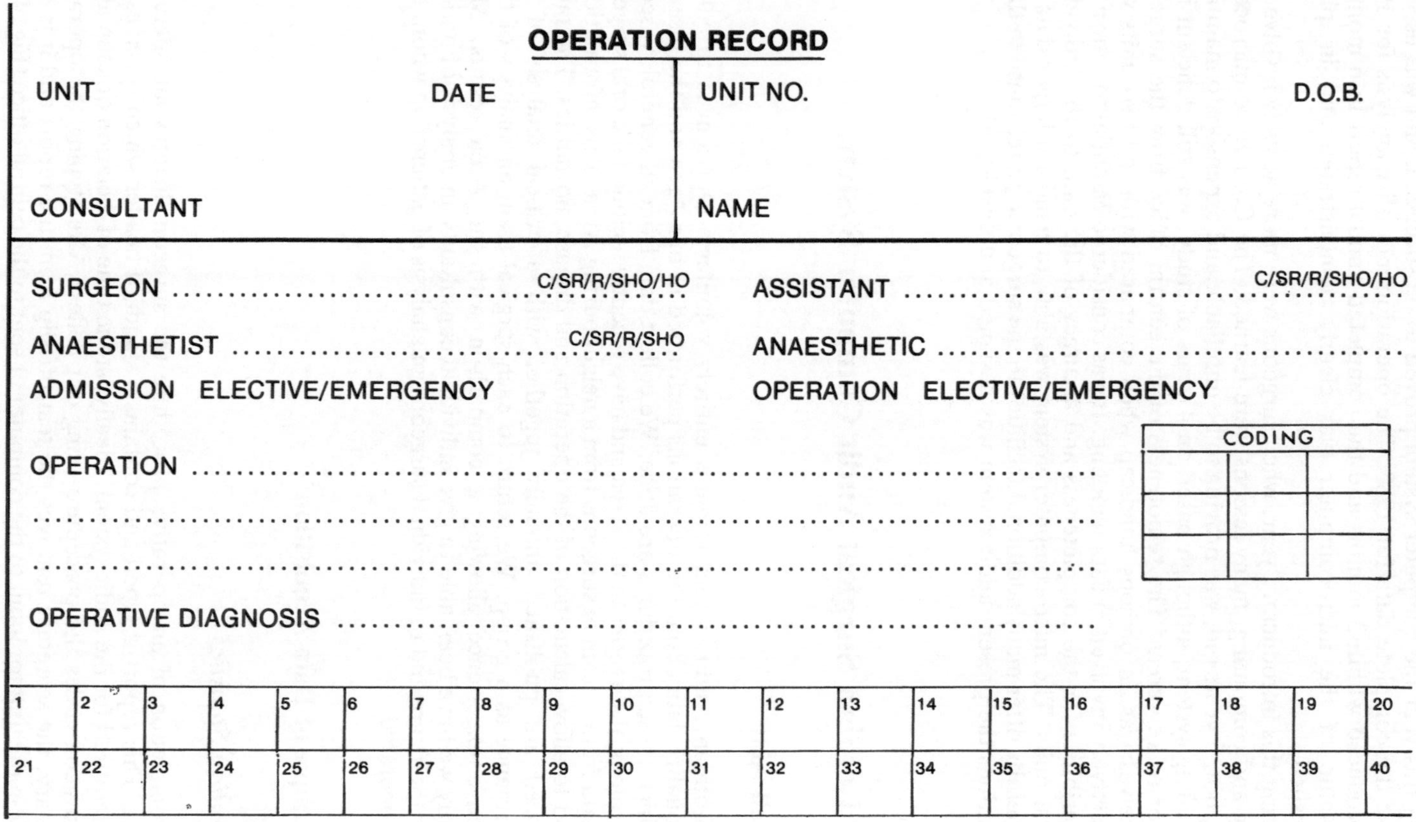

OPERATION RECORD

UNIT .... DATE .... UNIT NO. .... D.O.B. ....

CONSULTANT .... NAME ....

SURGEON .... C/SR/R/SHO/HO   ASSISTANT .... C/SR/R/SHO/HO

ANAESTHETIST .... C/SR/R/SHO   ANAESTHETIC ....

ADMISSION ELECTIVE/EMERGENCY   OPERATION ELECTIVE/EMERGENCY

OPERATION ....

OPERATIVE DIAGNOSIS ....

CODING

1	2	3	4	5	6	7	8	9	10	11	12	13	14	15	16	17	18	19	20
21	22	23	24	25	26	27	28	29	30	31	32	33	34	35	36	37	38	39	40

Fig. 4.1. Operation record.

During 1986 seven units entered their own data. Three surgical units have trained secretarial staff who have the responsibility of inputting data to a computer. Four surgical units have no such staff and the data entry is performed by junior medical staff. Surgeons in training are encouraged to code and enter their own data in order to grasp the fundamentals of acquiring high quality data. They are able to obtain analyses of their own work immediately the data is input and these documents are being increasingly used for training requirements and job applications. During 1986 the data from seven units have been entered centrally. For 1987 we have obtained further BBC Master systems so that six of these units will be able to enter their own data. In this way we have returned to the original concept that each unit would be responsible for its own data. Units now collect standardised and accurate data on a microcomputer which may be analysed individually or collectively.

We estimate that the total time required for data entry is one to two hours per week depending on the size of the data set and the experience of the user.

Choice of the Microcomputer and Hardware

In 1983 many low cost, home computers became available. We required a robust system that would stand professional use. A disc operating system capable of holding up to 3000 patient records per floppy disc with the possibility of expansion in the future was also essential. We foresaw that the introduction of microcomputers to surgical units would allow many other applications to be realised and that they would have considerable educational value. The recently introduced Acorn/BBC microcomputer seemed to fulfil our requirements and the initial programs were designed for this system. We have no reason to regret this decision and have now acquired seventeen complete BBC systems situated in seven hospitals throughout the Area. To date we have had no problems with reliability of these systems.

For our purposes the BBC computer has two major limitations. The maximum available RAM in BASIC is less than 30 K. This has presented few problems apart from the design of search and sort routines. The Disc Filing System (DFS) has a maximum file size of 200 K, the limit being set by the maximum possible file to be accommodated on one side of an 80-track, 5¼-inch floppy disc. Our audit system was designed for single drive use to keep costs low. The patient record length of 70 bytes limits the system to 2900 patient records per disc which is sufficient to store annual data for most of our surgical units. However, two surgical teams perform in excess of 5000 procedures per year and these units store data in 6-month periods. More recently we have acquired a number of BBC Master systems and are redesigning our programs to gain the advantages of the Advanced Disc Filing System which has unlimited file length and will accept a Winchester drive. We use a Master system in the central office with a 30 megabyte Winchester which now holds data on over 100 000 patient operations collected between 1983 and 1986.

The Acorn/BBC micro has many advantages which have proved to be of great value. We use the Teletext mode which offers the full range of 8 colours and yet has the maximum free RAM. The programs have been written in BBC BASIC using the structured features of this language. From the outset we have believed that a major factor in our work is the education of our colleagues in the use of this new technology. We have therefore written our programs in the computer language most likely to be learned by doctors. We have given all string and arithmetic variables names that indicate their function. The use of named procedures makes the programs easier to understand. Although BBC BASIC is fast enough for most uses we have been forced to employ machine code routines for sorting and searching. The availability of an assembler as standard in the BBC micros, together with the ease with which BASIC and machine code can be integrated into a single program have proved extremely valuable. The choice of the BBC computer also allowed interested doctors to use, study and develop the package of programs at home. As a result the present programs are understood by many of the junior hospital staff and the system is no longer dependent on the major author for future development.

As our system is essentially a database system it is relevant to ask why we have not used a commercial database package. In 1983 our intention was to produce a package which would simply store and count the operations performed annually by each surgical team. We did not envisage a more ambitious package that would include searching, listing, sorting etc. At that time there was no commercial system available for the BBC which could produce the types of analysis required. Programs to enter simple data are easily written in BASIC. More recently there has been a considerable improvement in commercial systems, although the simplicity of use and the quality of presentation we have been able to achieve is unlikely to have been produced by a commercial database system. We have been able to produce a system which few have managed to misuse. Our system does limit the number of records to 2900 if the sort and search programs are used. The data input, enquiry and analytic programs have no limit other than that of the file size limits of the disc-filing system. The use of a commercial package would have reduced much of the educational value of our system and would have added to the cost. Looking to the future, we may need to consider the use of a commercial system for basic data handling and complement this with utility programs for our special needs.

Since adopting the BBC microcomputer, our surgeons have developed many other applications including word processing. We have developed a statistical package which is widely used and the University Department of Medical Illustration has acquired the hardware to obtain high-quality photographic slides from the output of the BBC. The microcomputers have also been used for the diagnosis of acute abdominal pain, as Viewdata terminals and in the laboratory.

We provide medium-resolution colour monitors as we find that they are the minimum acceptable quality for word processing in 80-character mode. A dual, 80-track 5¼-inch disc drive and a low cost dot-matrix printer incorporating near-letter-quality print are provided with each system. At the time of writing the cost per unit is £1000.

Coding of Operations and Pathology

The coding system developed by our group is fundamental to the whole audit process. Most international codes have a pathological basis, but to a surgeon there are many clinical factors which are of considerable audit interest.

Examples are the presence of jaundice in biliary and pancreatic surgery, peritonitis in colo-rectal work and history of recent rupture in aortic aneurysm surgery. Many of these distinctions are not made in the ICD coding system. Similarly we found that the OPCS system for the classification of operations fell far short of the precision required. A system which does not distinguish important differences is unlikely to be accepted by medical staff nor is an unwieldy coding system of great complexity.

Our codes are based on a 3-number system, the first code indicating the organ, the second code specifying the pathological process and the third code giving the operation. This system has proved to be as precise as OPCS and ICD in two-thirds of operations and more precise in one-third of cases. There are 40 organ codes (recently increased to 51 with the inclusion of oral surgery). Each organ code has a unique list of appropriate pathologies and a list of operations. The programs allow for two further codes which increases definition if required. We have already employed the fourth code in cases of revision surgery (e.g. gastric surgery and amputation), indicating the nature of the previous operation. Vascular surgeons have used all five codes for vascular graft operations, the third code indicating the take-off point of the graft, the fourth indicating the termination of the graft and the fifth defining the nature of the graft (Dacron, reversed vein etc). These examples indicate that the coding system has proved flexible and able to cope with complex situations. The system is capable of extension in three distinct dimensions. The number of organ codes may be increased. The lists of pathologies and operations may be lengthened and finally the fourth and fifth codes may be employed. We are confident that our system will prove valuable for many years to come with only occasional minor revision.

We have attempted to analyse the accuracy of coding in a variety of ways. Twelve hundred slips from 12 units were re-coded and found to have a 3 % error. The major error was imprecision rather than an incorrect code. For example, a perforated duodenal ulcer may have been coded as a simple ulcer. The error rate is acceptably low. We have also attempted to analyse the completeness of the data. This has proved extremely difficult as no more accurate data source exists. We found that 5 % of operations which appear in the theatre book are not coded although the large majority of these are very minor procedures (e.g. rigid sigmoidoscopy, dressing changes etc) and obviously were not considered as operations by the surgical staff. Emergency procedures are more likely to be lost than elective procedures due to failure to dictate an operation report. Unit secretaries have a system to detect failure of dictation on elective surgical lists.

Description of the Patient Record and Data Files

Because of the limitations of the BBC DFS we have reserved one side of the 80-track disc (200 K) for patient data and use the other side for the programs and data files. Users of the BBC will be aware of the inability of the DFS to extend files once written. To avoid this problem a 200 K file, filling one side of the disc, is created at the beginning of each year and used subsequently.

The system has five data files summarised below.:

1. Main patient data file
2. Patient sort file
3. List of organs
4. List of pathologies
5. List of operations

Patient data are stored in ASCII files of fixed record length. All unallocated characters are stored as Hex 20 (32=space) to avoid any conflict on transfer of files to alternative microcomputers. Record 0 of the patient data file is unique in that it holds two numbers, the first being the record number (recordnumber%) of the next entry (this being incremented by one as each new operation statistic is entered) and the second being the record length (recordlength%). Each program initially reads these two numbers and sets pointers accordingly. Individual users may increase the record length to include new data by appending extra characters to each record and changing the value of recordlength%. All programs in the package will function normally after this simple change. The present record length is 70 bytes as shown below.

Hospital unit number	10
Organ code	2
Pathology code	2
Operation code	2
4th code	2
5th code	2
Emergency/elective flag	1
Multiple operation flag	1
Patient name	25
Mortality flag	1
Date of operation	6 (ddmmyy)
Consultant	4
Surgeon	4
Optional data	8
Total length	70

Ten digits are used for the unique hospital number. Two digits are available for each operation code (10 in all) allowing the numbering system to extend to 99. Emergency operations are flagged with the letter Y. Patient name is inserted with the surname first, all in upper case. The date of operation is recorded in standard style, day/month/year. Four characters are allowed to identify the consultant and surgeon. Eight optional characters are free for the user to insert personnel codes.

BBC BASIC can store data on disc in random access or sequential files. Patient data are stored using the random access technique which allows easy transfer of data between BBC, Cromemco and IBM PC systems. Random access is relatively slow. Data are read from and written to the disc one byte at a time (using the BGET and BPUT statements in BASIC). The slow speed is of little consequence during data entry but becomes more obvious in the analytical programs. Sequential access files in BBC BASIC store string variables backwards on disc and also include indicators of data type and length which would make transfer of data between computers more difficult.

The patient sort file contains the first five characters of each patient's name. This file is 15 K in length, containing up to 3000 names of patients, and may be loaded into RAM and rapidly searched to identify an individual patient. The technique is described more fully below.

The text of our coding system is held in three data files containing codes for organs, pathologies and operations. For simplicity and speed these are stored using a combination of the sequential and random-access techniques. Each new string is read and written using sequential data language (PRINT#, INPUT# statements in BASIC) but with the start of each string at regular intervals of 45 characters in the file. A pointer moves rapidly to the selected item and reads the file content. Empty records have been left throughout these files for future expansion of the system. Programs which use these datafiles include data statements pointing to the start records and number of records in the codes. Each year we have made additions to the coding system and this requires slight modification to the datafiles and a change in the pointers.

Additional files are generated by the programs themselves. The package includes programs to produce lists of patients in various orders (alphabetical, date order etc). These programs generate datafiles containing the record numbers in the appropriate order. Text files are produced during operation of analytical and search programs which may be read into a word-processing package (e.g. View) for subsequent editing. The creation of these files saves considerable secretarial time in producing final documents.

Description of the Programs

The audit package consists of a set of small BASIC programs each performing a limited task. In this way, individual programs may be easily debugged or replaced. Short programs also leave maximum RAM available to the programmer. I have not described each program in detail but have summarised the special problems presented in each of the programs and have described our solutions to these problems. The present package includes the following programs:

1. Data input
2. Search and modify data
3. Analysis of operation statistics
4. Detailed analysis of operation and pathology statistics
5. Specialised vascular graft analysis
6. Database enquiry
7. Listing of patients in specified order
8. Utilities

Data Input Program

As our system is entirely dependent on the cooperation of medical and secretarial staff it was felt that the programs had to be simple in operation and attractive to the eye. This is especially true of the program to enter the data. Full use has been made of the colour facilities of the BBC micro. Data are entered into colour-coded boxes. Two special procedures were written. The first was a simple routine to place a box of any colour and length in any specified position on the screen. This procedure is limited only by the line length of 40 characters in Teletext mode.

The second procedure allows data input within the confines of a box. The routine prevents the user from leaving the box except by pressing RETURN. Within a box it is possible to delete backwards but not outside the confines of the box. Only characters within a specified ASCII range are allowed. On pressing RETURN the resulting string is lengthened by addition of spaces (hex 20) to the correct length and stored. No word-processing ability within a box is present i.e. characters cannot be inserted or overwritten. This avoids the need for multiple commands to control the cursor.

The program moves from box to box in a circular fashion. After leaving a box, corrections may be made by returning to the box and re-typing the entry. By pressing RETURN the user is able to skip from box to box without altering the contents. As soon as an entry is made the program deletes the present contents of the box and inserts the new data.

The program does not include any check on the data. Errors of data entry occur but constitute a very small proportion of the total data entered. Error-checking routines are being developed which allow the user to define acceptable initials for the consultant and surgeon and which check dates. These are presently under test and may be included in future developments. It would be impossible to include routines to check names and codes. Checking routines are of undoubted value but the surgeons' commitment prevents most errors. Prior to publishing annual unit reports the detailed printouts are carefully examined and obvious coding errors corrected.

The TAB key is used to indicate that data entry is complete and the record is written to disc. The position of the record in the file is obtained from record 0 of the patient file, the pointer is moved to the correct position and the patient record string is written.

Search and Modify Data

We did not intend this system to be used to find individual patient records, but we soon found that this was needed. Each patient record is allocated a computer number, that is, the position in the patient datafile. An individual record may be rapidly located and displayed if this number is known. In practice, a clinician is more likely to know a patient's name. A BASIC program was written which would search the patient data file record by record. It could take up to 2 minutes to find the 2000th record, too slow for regular use.

We adopted an alternative technique in which a special file was created containing the first five characters of each patient's name in the same order as in the main datafile. This file could be loaded into RAM and searched. If a match was found then the remainder of the name was read from the disc and compared. This technique in BASIC was able to locate the 2000th record in 24 seconds, the rate-limiting factor being the BASIC search of memory. The logical progression was to replace the BASIC memory search with a small machine-code routine. The resulting package is able to search through 3000 patients in less than 1 second. There is no appreciable delay in the location of a record if given a patient's name when compared with the delay if the computer is given the exact position of the patient in the datafile. Whilst the available memory space limits this technique to a search of 3000 patients, this may be increased by using fewer than five characters of each patient's name. Alternatively, the recent introduction of HI–BASIC for the BBC Master increases available RAM and would allow a further expansion to 9000 patients.

Having located a patient by computer number or name any field of data may be changed by using the data-entry program. The sort file is constantly updated during operation of the data-entry or search programs. A utility program will recreate the sort file if it becomes corrupted.

Analysis of Operation Statistics

Two levels of statistical analysis are used. The simpler of the two programs counts the number of operations of each type performed for a named consultant, a named surgeon or of the whole data set.

Although there are 40 organ codes in our system there are only 23 lists of operations as some organs share a common list e.g. oesophagus/stomach/duodenum. There are up to 99 operations in each list. A complete analysis including mortality and distinction between emergency and elective operations would require a data array of $23 \times 100 \times 2 \times 2 = 9200$ separate items, far in excess of the capability of the BBC microcomputer. Using the technique of masking it is possible to store more than one piece of numerical data in a single number. For example, if there were 129 emergency appendicectomies and 21 elective appendicectomies in one year this could be expressed as the single integer 129021 where the thousands indicate emergency operations and the single digits the elective cases. By using this technique we have been able to analyse elective/emergency data in a single pass but require a second pass to analyse mortality.

A typical example of the summary analysis for one organ (hernia) is shown in Table 4.1. The mortality data are added later.

This program will analyse the workload of one consultant, one surgeon or the whole unit combined. The table may be printed or stored as a text file. A complete analysis at this level with 2000 procedures takes 5 minutes.

Detailed Analysis of Operation and Pathology Statistics

The summary described above used only two of the three codes in our system i.e. organ and operation. A more detailed analysis is possible if the pathology code is also included. The data array would now increase to $40 \times 100 \times 100 \times 2 \times 2 = 1\,600\,000$ elements. Multiple passes are avoided by storing

Table 4.1   A summary analysis for hernia

Emergency	Elective	Total	Mortality	
33	831	864	(5)	Inguinal hernia (+/− orchidectomy)
5	112	117		Recurrent inguinal
35	58	93	(4)	Femoral
0	3	3		Recurrent femoral
12	80	92		Incisional
0	8	8		Recurrent incisional
10	42	52		Para-umbilical
5	27	32		Epigastric
0	2	2		Spigelian
1	3	4		Other

only those code combinations which actually occur. As data are read from each patient the program checks the operation code against those already stored. If a new procedure is encountered then the program stores the new code. As the list of codes increases in length the program runs more slowly. The program ranks the codes in ascending order prior to printing the result. The program is able to print a detailed analysis of 2000 patients in less than 10 minutes and, like the previous program, may be tailored to analyse the whole data set or the work of a specified surgeon. Table 4.2 gives, as an example, a more detailed analysis of hernia data than Table 4.1.

Table 4.2   A detailed analysis of hernia data

Elective	Emergency	Total	Mortality	
Simple				
6	809	815	(2)	Inguinal
0	110	110		Recurrent inguinal
2	44	46		Femoral
0	3	3		Recurrent femoral
2	72	74		Incisional
0	7	7		Recurrent incisional
Irreducible				
12	15	27		Inguinal
2	1	3		Recurrent inguinal
13	8	21	(2)	Femoral
4	6	10		Incisional
0	1	1		Recurrent incisional
Obstructed				
13	5	18	(1)	Inguinal
3	1	4		Recurrent inguinal
12	3	15		Femoral
4	2	6		Incisional
Gangrenous (requiring resection)				
1	1	2	(1)	Inguinal
8	2	10	(2)	Femoral
1	0	1		Incisional

Vascular Graft Analysis Programs

Our vascular surgeons have increased the complexity of the coding which has required modification of the programs. The programs are similar and are not described further.

Database Enquiry

This program allows the user to print a list of patients with a specified pathology or operation and is used for the generation of lists to allow retrospective studies. For complex searches the user may separately define seven search criteria in one pass. Each search pattern requires a specified organ, up to five defined pathologies and up to five defined operations. For example, to list all patients undergoing surgery for Crohn's disease would require three search criteria, the organs being small bowel, colo-rectum and peri-anal. Only one pathology is required for small bowel and colo-rectum but three pathology codes are used to distinguish perianal Crohn's disease. The search criteria would appear as listed in Table 4.3.

Table 4.3. Search criteria to identify all patients in the data file with Crohn's disease

Organ	Pathology	Operation
5 (Small bowel)	5	All
7 (Colo-rectum)	10	All
8 (Perianal)	8,9,10	All

This complex search pattern would require only a single pass through the data and all relevant records would be printed in full. The program is able to scan 2000 patients in under 5 minutes. The user may specify an individual consultant or surgeon and the resulting list may be printed or stored as a text file. The program has no particular special features and is not limited other than by the size of the datafile. The list of patients is printed in the order of insertion but we intend to merge this program with the "sorting" programs described below to allow the lists to be printed in a variety of orders (alphabetical, date etc).

Listing of Patients in Specified Order

The listing of patients in various orders may be useful. A suite of programs has been written to list patients alphabetically, by date order, operation code order and hospital number. No attempt is made to sort records as data are entered. At any time, the records input so far may be ordered. During the development of these programs the sort technique employed has been progressively improved for greater speed and flexibility. Sorting is performed in memory by reading the relevant part of each record (up to 6 characters) into RAM and using two adjacent bytes to store the original record number. The records are then sorted and the record number passively exchanged in any swop. On completion of the sort, the record numbers (now in sorted order) are saved to disc and this file is used to move the pointer within the main patient datafile as the sorted list is printed. During execution, the main datafile is not modified in any way.

Initially a simple bubble sort was employed but this was much too slow when the number of records exceeded 1000. Some improvement was gained with a shell-sort technique but this was replaced by a recursion routine. This BASIC routine was capable of sorting 2000 records in less than 3 minutes. A considerable quantity of RAM was required limiting the program to 2000 records. Recently we have used a machine-code bubble sort capable of sorting 2000 records in 4 minutes and 3000 records in 8 minutes. By using HI–BASIC this routine may be able to sort 9000 records although the time taken may prove excessive. Future developments may increase this speed.

The same sort routine is applicable to all four sorting programs although sorting by date requires that the dates be reversed (yymmdd) as they are read into memory. Patient names and hospital numbers are sorted by the first 6 characters. The routines have been written in such a way that the lengths of the strings used in the sort may be varied easily and a small data set could be sorted by name using all 25 characters if required. The routines could be modified to allow sorting on multiple fields but this has not proved necessary.

Utility Programs

During the development of the package a number of utility programs have been written. These include programs to create a new database and to back-up the datafiles. There is a program to generate age distributions and to allow more rapid correction of data, as some units initially entered patient names in the incorrect order. With many doctors using the same datafile we find that initials of surgeon and consultant may vary and a utility is available which will list all initials used in a database and correct any errors. A utility program will extract all records of one consultant or one surgeon and create a separate database for individual use. These small programs are available to users on request.

Discussion

When considering the value of a package of computer programs, the view of the writer on its success is no more to be believed than the view of a surgeon on how successful his operations are. With that in mind the following comments on the success of our system must be read with some suspicion.

If we have succeeded then much of that success is due to our unique circumstances. We have been fortunate in that a manual system of data collection has existed for more than 40 years in our Area. Our surgeons have been prepared openly to discuss workloads and surgical mortality with their colleagues. All surgical teams have a desire to collect structured, high quality data and have been prepared to spend the necessary time and effort in obtaining these data voluntarily. Especially valuable has been the development of a coding system for diseases and operations based on experience of more than 200 000 operations between 1978 and 1986. During this period, a system of data collection from operation reports was developed and a structured mortality data sheet was devised. We have also been extremely fortunate that a small group of surgeons and community medical specialists have been prepared to devote much of their time and effort to the development of the audit system. Recently, many of our junior hospital doctors have developed an interest in microcomputer techniques and our work has been supported financially by research funds and the Lothian Health Board.

The proof of the success of a database system must be the quantity, quality and completeness of the data collected and the use to which it is put. At the present time we have computer data concerning over 100 000 operations performed over a 4-year period. The data have been derived from 8 hospitals, 15 teams of surgeons and more than 30 consultants with their junior staff. We estimate that the data are 95 % complete and 97 % accurate. Our major aim is to identify areas of surgery where morbidity and mortality are high and to encourage further study of these areas. We believe that we have made a significant contribution to the critical examination of our performance as surgeons and have influenced changes in practice.

We believe that the conclusions drawn from comparison of results of surgery in general and in specialised units has been a factor in formation of urological and vascular units in our Area. In the same way, general surgeons have abandoned certain operations in favour of their specialist colleagues whose results are better. We have undertaken detailed reviews of the results following colo-rectal operations and surgery for upper gastro-intestinal haemorrhage which have led to prospective clinical trials and changes in practice. A prospective study of radiotherapy in oesophageal cancer was initiated following audit work. These are tangible results of our audit process but we believe that we have stimulated an on-going self-audit amongst our surgical colleagues which is contributing to the improved results of surgery.

Our data are used annually to generate a detailed report of the operative workload and mortality of each contributing unit and the combined analysis of the Area. These reports have been published in the spring of the following year and discussed at surgical meetings. These data have been extensively used by our surgical colleagues for lectures at undergraduate and postgraduate levels and have often provided the stimulus for retrospective studies. This use of our data is growing as more surgeons realise the value of our data sets in identifying patients with particular diseases and specific operations. All individual units have immediate access to their own data for the period 1983–86. Any request for lists of patients is passed to all relevant consultants for permission to study patients under their care. To date, no such request has been refused.

Surgeons in training increasingly use our data to quantify operative experience and training committees at registrar and senior registrar level have adopted our codes for collection of data. The data have also been used for work study in discussions of the provision of facilities and man-power planning.

During the 4-year period of microcomputer development we have been able to overcome many hurdles and refute many previous arguments concerning the use of computers in patient data analysis. Certainly we have shown that a low-cost microcomputer is capable of handling a very large, and growing, data set. Our present 30 megabyte BBC system should be sufficient for our needs over the next 5 years unless we extend the data set considerably. We have had no problems with the reliability of our BBC systems and have suffered no serious loss of data throughout this period.

Our programs have been entirely written by medical staff with support from the Health Board computing staff. We have therefore been able to demonstrate that large data sets may be acquired at very low cost and with little expertise and formal training. Our initial decision to write our own database system was forced upon us by circumstance. Future developments might well benefit from the use of a commercial system but the educational value of such a system would be considerably less than we have achieved.

We have found that medical staff are eager to adopt new technology and have welcomed the introduction of microcomputers. Accepting that our colleagues are already highly trained and motivated, none-the-less they have rapidly learned to use our package and many have made significant contributions to its further development. Our junior staff have been prepared to input many of the data to computer, being attracted by the immediate recall and analysis programs of the package. Contrary to general belief, our doctors have been prepared to code their own operations. This is fundamental to our work as the data collected by our system belong to the surgeons themselves. The analyses are therefore the surgeon's own opinion of the nature of the disease processes and the type of operations performed rather than a coding clerk's interpretation of a registrar's discharge letter. We believe that our surgeons have accepted the task of coding partly because of the simplicity and speed of our coding system and also because they realise that it offers a very accurate and precise basis for data collection.

As our basic data set has increased the question of data confidentiality has arisen. In fact the data we collect is no more detailed than that collected centrally for hospital in-patient statistics. Our data are more freely accessible to the individual, more up-to-date and much more accurate than the centralised data set. Our operation statistics are also comparable to those recorded in theatre books. There is a dilemma between the need to maintain confidentiality and the need to allow easy entry and use of the system. We make no attempt to limit entry to the system as we encourage all surgical staff to use the system. As we are concerned to educate our colleagues in the use of computers it would seem pointless to devise protection techniques which would act as a stimulus to unravel the protection. We have registered in accordance with the Data Protection Act and have found this Act to be of great value. The data that we collect belong to the surgeons and we do not produce any analysis without their expressed consent. We make clear to our colleagues and administration that analysis of data without consent of individuals concerned is illegal and will not be undertaken.

The Lothian Surgical Audit has developed over many years. It has been described as creeping evolution, with small but significant improvements made each year. We still collect a very limited data set but we have managed to maintain the involvement and interest of all of our colleagues. The recent introduction of microcomputers to all the contributing units offers new and exciting possibilities. We may be able to integrate our system into the day-to-day running of the surgical units and hope to develop waiting-list, operation-report and discharge-letter facilities. In this way we would be able to generate accurate audit reports as a by-product of our routine work. We intend to expand into the field of morbidity by collecting defined data from the whole Area over a short period and so produce a snapshot of aspects of morbidity such as wound infection, chest infection etc. By this technique we hope to identify areas of morbidity where improvements should be sought. We have also received requests from other specialties including oral surgery, orthopaedics and gastro-intestinal endoscopy to join our system.

Many surgeons, and small groups, have described the use of microcomputer-based systems for surgical audit. However, we know of no similar system of mortality audit which has been adopted by all relevant surgeons of an Area Health Authority. Our work has clearly shown the willingness of surgical colleagues to cooperate in the collection of high-quality audit data on computer and the capability of microcomputers to provide a valuable clinical service. Future developments to include out-patient planning, the production of waiting-lists, letter writing etc will require substantial financial support and professional computing advice. However, our limited project has provided surgeons with both valuable data and experience in computing methods.

We have freely given our coding systems and computer programs to any surgeons interested in the development of a similar operation/mortality audit.

Summary

A microcomputer-based system has been developed to analyse operation and mortality statistics collected voluntarily by general, urological, vascular and oral surgeons in the Lothian Region of Scotland. The system collects data on 25 000 operations annually and over 400 deaths. It currently holds data on over 100 000 operations. A unique coding system of disease and operations has been devised which offers more detail than the ICD/OPCS systems combined and yet is simpler to use. Medical staff perform the coding. The complete package is able to analyse operation statistics for the whole Area, for surgical teams and for individual consultants and surgeons. We have been able to acquire a computer system for each surgical unit. We believe that our work has led to significant changes in clinical practice. The introduction of microcomputers throughout the Area has proved highly successful not only for audit but also in the education of our medical and secretarial colleagues in computer techniques and in the development of many alternative applications.

Acknowledgements

I would like to thank the many surgeons in the Lothian Area of Scotland who contributed to our audit and especially those members of the Surgical Audit Committee. Particular mention is made of Dr R. Gruer and Mr C.V. Ruckley for their work in the initial development of the audit system and Mr A.A. Gunn for help with development of the codes and his valuable advice and support. I acknowledge the continuing support of the Lothian Health Board Edinburgh.

5 The Development of a Distributed Surgical Audit System

J.R. Coughlan, M.J. Taylor, W.A. Corbett and R. Shields

There is a need [1] for the collection and analysis of information concerning clinical workload and performance. The information resulting from the analysis of patterns and trends with the raw patient record data is a valuable tool for the improved management of both patients and the resources available [2].

The need for up-to-date and accurate information has been recognised within the top levels of management in the National Health Service (NHS). From the point of view of the administrator, as opposed to the clinician, targets have been set by the reports of Korner and Griffiths [3,4]. The spending of the NHS on information technology is low, on both hardware and staffing counts, relative to other organisations. This, together with the tight controls on its direction from Regional Health Authorities (RHA) remote from the day-to-day management of hospital patients, has not inspired the confidence of clinical staff to believe that they will be provided with systems of immediate first-hand value.

Many hospitals, including the Royal Liverpool, serve a given department with one terminal for data input to a remote main-frame. This is provided almost solely for the input of out-patient data by clerical staff, although limited queries based on searches under an individual name or case-sheet number are sometimes possible. Additionally, a manually collected form of summarised hospital throughput has evolved, known as the Hospital Activity Analysis. Although providing some guide to numbers, the system has several limitations which involve incomplete and insufficiently specific data, and as the interval between data collection and production of reports is long (more than 8 months in our particular case) such reports have diminished relevance by the time they filter back to the clinical level.

Given the need to base changes in internal management strategies upon accurate and timely information, this department has conducted an audit examining the throughput and care of its patients. In the case of the Department of Surgery, a formal paper-based method has been in use for the past 10 years whereby the junior doctors are responsible for collecting, summarising and presenting a limited selection of data concerning overall activities within the department during a three-month period. In gross terms, this gives an indication of the quantity e.g. number of operations performed, and quality e.g. wound infection rates, of the departmental workload, which can be broken down by individual members of staff. By examining the results for different quarterly periods, with adjustment for seasonal factors, clinical problems can be highlighted and attention focused on surgical strategies, admissions routines and prescription policies, which are reviewed and changed where necessary at the regular departmental meetings called for this purpose.

Although of far more use than the centralised reports referred to previously, the volume of data (from approximately 500 patients), and hence the time taken to look through all the paper containing it, mean that the 3-monthly reports can only be compiled on a limited, pre-defined basis, with little cross-tabulating or itemising of the first-order data apart from those of obvious interest or relevance such as patients who developed wound infections or who died while under the care of the Department.

System Requirements

It had been clear for some time that the interests of greater accuracy, and more sophisticated analyses over varying time periods could only be served by the introduction of a computer-based system for both data collection and report generation. Preferable solutions would include the capacity for ad-hoc queries and, more importantly, would bring the maximum benefits for busy staff with minimal disruption to their normal routine. Additionally, it was felt then any such system would have to be designed and operated solely by the Department, to ensure sufficient control over its form and function.

It was felt important that data collection should be driven by and follow the known patterns of data flow within the Department. These can be thought of as the movement of incomplete records on patients involved with the Department from one list to another, each list being a grouping of records of similar levels of completion (Fig. 5.1). The normal sequential and chronological flow would be from the waiting list that patients are placed on after attendance at clinic, through the admissions list, expected list and ward list, to the discharge list on leaving hospital. This holds for the majority of patients, who are treated on an elective basis. Exceptions obviously occur, and must be catered for, both in the case of emergency admissions direct to the wards, and those elective patients who are unable to come in when first expected.

The known problems of missing and incorrect data were thought to be best eliminated by making the partially completed records the source of reference for clerical and clinical staff wherever possible. Any additions and changes would thus be immediately obvious to staff who would have the correct details in mind at the time. This would also obviate the persistent duplication, with its attendant scope for the introduction of errors, of the same items of data collected via a number of paper forms. The incentive to busy staff to run a system requiring

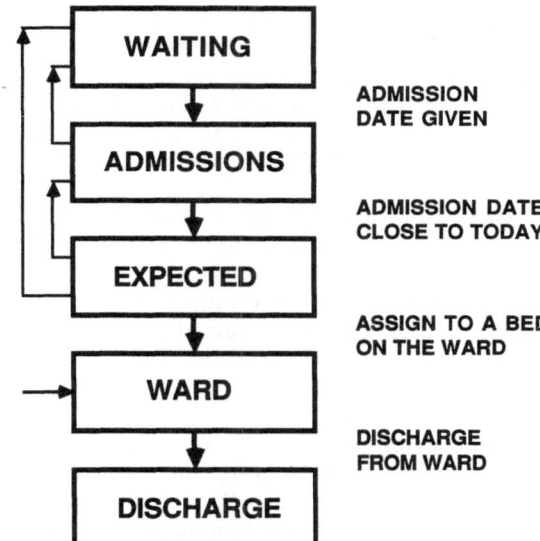

Fig. 5.1. Transaction flow paths.

such timely input of data would be to furnish the system with the capabilities to assist with the mainly clerical manipulations normally performed from the paper records, for example, the generation of admission lists and operation lists. The individual case notes would still have to be maintained but it was planned that discharge summaries could be produced for direct insertion into the case notes after being signed as correct by the relevant responsible clinician, together with a similar discharge letter for the patient's general practitioner.

In short, it was felt that only by integrating the collection of data with its use and manipulation within the Department could we be sure of gathering information of the quality needed. This implied a system based more on active office automation principles than on passive data collection after the events. At a more general level, other qualities required of the system were for it to be robust, with good error-recovery procedures, easy for staff to use, with a minimum of training required (important because of staff turnover), of lowest possible cost, and with the capability to withstand expansion and upgrade changes.

Design Solutions

The use of a commercially available off-the-shelf database package would save considerably on programming effort. The software packages examined all had severe limitations of one form or another, either in the cost of the machine required to run them, or in their intrinsic abilities.

On looking at the available solutions it was seen that there were three main variants.

A Single-Site, Single-User Microcomputer. This would have been both the most economical and the simplest system to implement. However, it was considered that as it would still need the intermediary of paper records, it would only serve to computerise the existing omissions and inaccuracies, as well as being of little use to staff in differing locations. The similar option of using an existing terminal to the university main-frame had the additional drawbacks of restricted or expensive software and concern over the protection of the data from unauthorised interference.

A Multi-User Minicomputer with Several Terminals. Such a system is an expensive option, even though it would have gone some way towards a solution to the problems, but given that the RHA was itself contemplating providing equipment for the same nominal purpose, it would have been difficult, if not impossible, to raise the required finance. There were also doubts as to whether the screen generators and input routines of the commercial databases available were sufficiently powerful and flexible for our needs.

A Microcomputer Network. A microcomputer network solution was adopted based on a central machine and microcomputer workstations. Funding indicated, however, that once the central machine and its associated software had been purchased the outlying microcomputers would have to be of a very low unit cost. A major drawback of the proposal, the increased development time due to the need to connect equipment and software from more than one manufacturer, was accepted in the light of what was possible from a financial viewpoint. By using distributed workstations, it was also intended to carry out research into the provision of task-orientated screens by way of a data-capture program to assist the user with data input; the benefit of this was the ability to validate such input as far as possible during its original entry before its incorporation into the database proper.

The Solution

The relational database management system, Informix, is run under the Xenix operating system, on an IBM PC-compatible Compaq Deskpro fitted with a 30 Mbyte hard disc [5,6]. Completed patient records are taken up into the database; those still in use are held in text files corresponding to the various lists. A file serving program, multi-tasked with the database, passes these files out to, and receives them back from the workstations, via an RS232-based Local Area Network, Infaplug [7]. The workstations, Sinclair QLs with memories expanded to 512 K, run the counterpart of the file transfer program, a real-time clock display program, and the data-capture program itself. A small BASIC program oversees the operation of the workstation software as a whole, all of which, together with any datafiles present, are held on RAM discs within the QL.

The System Centre

The primary requirements for the system centre were a good database management system that would run alongside a file-serving package, under a secure multi-tasking operating system, on a machine with sufficient storage capacity. At first it was thought that a Sinclair QL could be pressed into service, but doubts about the hard discs available, and the speed and flexibility of the database software, particularly with regard to entering data from external files rather than the keyboard, soon emerged togther with the wider considerations of possible future upgrades and the implications of a non-standard operating system. The BBC model B and other similar machines were eliminated on the grounds of limited capabilities, the most obvious symptom of which, rendering them unfit for our purposes, was their inability to support a true multi-tasking operating system. Machines running either MSDOS or CP/M were a little better in that they could offer databases more consonant with requirements, yet they too fell short of the multi-tasking role.

Thus we selected the Unix derivative, Xenix, to run on an IBM PC or compatible. This offers the desirable additional features of password controlled operations and the ability to execute pre-assigned tasks at given times without the need for the user to be logged on. As this was likely to be a standard in operating systems for a wide range of machines no problems were envisaged in later upgrades.

The host machine chosen, a Compaq Deskpro, had several advantages over the standard IBM machine available at the time of purchase. These included a more powerful processor, more RAM (640 K) for no extra cost, a larger capacity hard disc (30 Mbyte), and the option of a tape cartridge drive for fast back-ups.

The database, Informix, was chosen once it had been established that it was capable of the functions required i.e. multi-tasking and the capability to lift data from disc files. It has several important attributes in addition to the normal screen generator, report writer and interactive query language. These include an English-like programming language, full relational abilities, compilation of routines for fast execution, and a menu-driven front-end that can be customised for individual users. Additional permission settings may be applied to different users to allow differential access for insertions, alterations and deletions to the same datafile.

Unix and its derivatives have been criticised by some as being incomprehensible to inexperienced users, but it is often left unmentioned that they have the power to set up and present to such users any desired interface upon logging in. In the Department, users are required to do nothing more complicated than to press a single key or to enter dates to prompts in order to use most of the menu selections offered. These selections are not restricted to Informix functions; system back-up can be performed, for example, and other options to the menus can easily be added as the menu items themselves are held in an Informix database.

For surgical audit purposes, there are two main datafiles, the main one for admissions, linked to the second file, with subsidiary files which contain the accepted abbreviations for the common operations and diagnoses encountered within the departmental workload, along with their given World Health Organisation codings. These subsidiary files have three main functions: the generation of menu text files (described under workstations); look-up tables for diagnosis and operation entries; WHO Coding look-ups for activity summaries for the RHA.

A number of patients admitted to the Department are entered into various clinical trials. Using the relational capabilities of the database it is possible to provide separate menu driver screens and files for additional data entry which link with the standard data set collected for all patients.

One of the most important functions of any database is the provision of reports summarising its contents in one form or another. Currently there are over thirty standard reports on offer to the user. These include simple "how many of each type", cross-tabulations of several fields, reports written to fulfil standard defined surgical audit queries, and those designed to show up patterns in the data, for example, those operations where patients are found to have stayed on the ward for longer than expected. Several reports feature analysis of second-order data derived from the original, i.e. calculations involving the mean differences between the two date fields (Table 5.1). Reports are selected from a menu of their titles, the user enters the starting and finishing admission dates for the desired analysis, is shown the resulting output at the screen and is given an option for it to be printed, before being returned to the menus.

Table 5.1. Length of post-operative recovery time in days, listed by consultant. Report generated at 17:50:26 on 14/01/87, for patients admitted between 01/08/86 and 31/10/86 and subjected to a surgical procedure

Consultant	No. of procedures	% of procedures	Minimum recovery time	Maximum recovery time	Mean recovery time	Total bed day usage
A	36	13.58	1	14	4.06	146
B	89	33.58	0	14	3.09	275
C	94	35.47	0	36	4.11	386
D	46	17.36	1	61	8.59	395
Total	265	100.00	0	61	4.54	1202

Should a new type of request arise, there are three main options for the user:

1. Edit an existing report source file and recompile it if the differences are slight
2. Make up a completely new report, and compile it
3. If the query is one-off and relatively simple, use the interactive query language facility, although the command sequences used in this may be saved and re-applied if required

Some of the reports have been written to check the database for errors and inconsistencies, the order of dates being particularly important. A check for suspected duplicate records is done, although unique indexing normally rejects these upon data entry.

Browsing is normally performed through the generated screens, a system of "master and detail" file designations making it easy to connect from one file to another while doing so. Query by forms, where a blank form is completed with the search requirements, is a very useful feature for the naive user.

At all times there is the opportunity of directing output to a disc text file. Having done this, the resulting file may be used as the raw input for a word processor, or written out to a floppy disc for movement to another machine. One particular use is to transfer datafiles to the university IBM main-frame, for further statistical analysis and/or graphical representation.

For the uptake of completed patient records from their disc file, a small C utility routine has been written to convert the flat form of the QL records into two text files of the form and field ordering specified by the database. An overall command script, triggered by the existence of completed records, activates both this utility and the database load procedure.

The present Compaq [6] is insufficient to support more than one user, but upgrading to another Xenix/Unix machine would involve little more than bringing across the existing data and recompiling the source texts for the various routines already developed. In the future a more powerful computer may be purchased to service departmental needs, including database handling and word processing, leaving the Compaq to gather the data for analysis on the larger machine.

Inter-Machine File Transfer

Having decided to implement a system based on the movement of files between a central machine and a number of workstations, we examined the mechanisms available for doing so. Most of the commercially available solutions, such as those based on add-on cards for IBM PC compatibles, or datafiles to the university IBM main-frame, were discarded directly on the basis that the costs of both their intrinsic hardware and available host machine requirements far exceeded the budget.

We accepted that we would lose the fast transfer rates possible with that technology, and would have to reduce transmission to a level dictated by the speeds possible with standard asynchronous RS232 ports and the capability of the processor to control the file transfer mechanism. This last aspect was important, for although a wire link may connect two machines, substantial control and monitoring of the traffic is necessary for anything more involved than terminal emulation of one on the other. Additionally, we were looking for a system with the overall potential to handle the set-up of connections, transmission of files, and any associated error recovery procedures, on a completely automatic basis over long periods of time. One further complication was that as the hard-wired control lines on the Compaq serial ports did not appear to be controlled by Xenix as expected, we would have to use the XON/XOFF software protocols on this machine. Such control was not available on the QL except at baud rates low enough to allow user software to provide them. Hence the requirement was for a system able to connect different micros using different flow control mechanisms, and possibly differing baud rates as well.

There were only a few local area networks that appeared to meet our requirements and Infaplug was selected because it utilises plugs containing the active network electronics placed into cheap passive sockets on the cable ring. This allows a plug to be moved from socket to socket without disruption of the network. It also means that a faulty plug will not cause the remainder of the network to fail since it may be removed from its socket. The plugs have a wide range of internal options to enable communication with their assigned machine and, by translating inter-machine messages into their own proprietary protocol for transmission around the ring, each connected machine can use the options found most appropriate. The control codes needed to set up and clear network connections could easily be provided by a straightforward piece of software. The network could also be used to drive stand-alone printers. Finally, the plugs contain a "queueing" option to stack incoming calls if they have not yet completed the current one. The geographical layout of the network is shown in Fig. 5.2.

The Infaplug manufacturers had a user-driven package to run under the MSDOS operating system alone. We had either to write our own package, or to obtain other software that would serve as a basis for development to our requirements. Source code from the public domain file Kermit is now run, in modified forms, on both the Compaq and the QL workstations.

The basis of packet-exchange file transfer protocols such as Kermit [8], is that the connected machines send small blocks of bytes, the packets, to each other, proceeding to their next stage on the basis of obtaining the acknowledgement (or lack of one) from the receiving machine. Examples of such packets, which are all of similar basic structure within a single protocol, are the acknowledgement packets, control packets to determine the parameters to be used during a transfer, and the data packets themselves.

When a file is sent by Kermit a number of bytes consonant with the maximum packet length are read from the file into a packet, which is subject to a checksum analysis, the result of which is also placed in the packet before transmission. Upon receipt, the opposing machine removes the data from the packet, performs its own checksum and compares the result with that received in the packet. If there are no discrepancies, the data are copied to the destination file and an ACKNOWLEDGEMENT packet returned, otherwise a NOT ACK-NOWLEDGED packet is transmitted. Retransmissions and timeouts allow the protocol to persevere over noisy lines, which introduce random transmission errors, while other routines outside the general transmission protocol permit the package to interface with the machine hosting it.

Versions of Kermit were available for a number of machines and their associated operating systems; but not, unfortunately, for the QL. The C

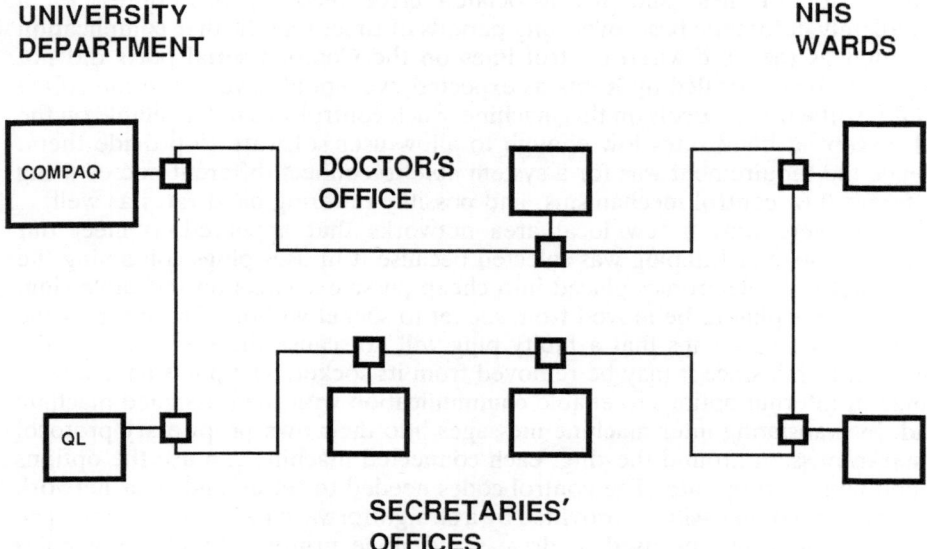

Fig. 5.2. Network layout.

language Unix version source was obtained for the Compaq, and as a base from which to produce a new version for the QL. The Unix Kermit as it came had many with useful features. Some of these have been removed to reduce the size of the code, for example the modem support routines. Specific additions then had to be designed and incorporated for our purpose, the main intention of which was to produce a file server controlled totally by the QL workstations requesting or sending a given file. These additions include a means of verifying the user name and password provided by a would-be workstation operator, and an internal file status table which prevents the same file being issued to more than one workstation at a time. They also facilitate recovery from the situation of one or more files not being returned within a given time limit, for whatever reason.

The action of the data-capture program may be viewed conceptually as working on an intake of one or more files of lists to produce similar files as output, after the possible movement of records between the various lists. If the destination list is currently held in the same QL, then simple overwriting will serve as an update when the files arrive back at the Compaq. There will be occasions, however, when one or more records are split off with the intention that they should join a list not currently present in the workstation, but possibly held by another QL or just dormant in the file server. These new files are returned under their normal names, and by inspection of the file status table, in conjunction with knowing the current sender's user name, the server program can take the correct decision with regard to appending the incoming file to its namesake, or holding it in a temporary file for later appendage to the original when it is returned by another workstation.

On the QL much more work was involved to implement file transfer. The original source was written in a version of C with many references to the Unix operating system. Substitutes for these were written, approximately half of the original features and functions removed as being superfluous, and new routines inserted to control the plugs and verify passwords. The advantage of having the source code for a defined protocol is that new packet types and the appropriate responses to them can be added, as has been done. The file transfers in the system were to be completely automated, freeing the users of the responsibility for fetching and returning datafiles. This meant writing into the QL Kermit the ability to be driven by commands from one or more nominated external files, and a substantial capacity to survive and continue to provide service on encountering error conditions. This last includes timeouts on all operations, and the ability to indicate that a particular transfer was unsuccessful while proceeding with the next.

In operation Kermit on the Compaq is run as a continual background task, in permanent server mode, driven by the incoming packets from the QL workstations. In a typical session on these, once the required batch of files has been nominated by the user, the QL Kermit attempts to connect through to the Compaq. It may succeed first time, or be placed in the call queue. When the connection is established, and the user identity confirmed, the request packets are serviced where possible, and the connection cleared to permit the next call to go through. Following the completion of data entry, the same procedure is repeated to return the files.

It was decided that data should be transmitted across the network in the form of ASCII files, whatever its optimal representation in the individual machines.

Although loading and saving record images would be more rapid than their reconstruction from text files, in the system as a whole other disadvantages would be evident. The main disadvantage would be that the transmission of a pseudo-binary file through the Kermit protocols involves flagging each non-ASCII character to indicate its nature to the receiver. The consequent increase in network transfer time for such files would far outweigh any savings made in loading and saving, which are not slow as the files are held on RAM discs. Another consideration is that should such a file of records be damaged, it would be a simple matter to repair with a text editor. It was also uncertain whether or not the plugs and the two operating systems involved could be completely shielded from a chance encounter with a binary sequence normally used to exert a control signal. Such a philosophy may not be tenable in large-scale commercial systems, but here we are dealing with small numbers of small files.

The Workstations

The requirements for these were exacting; the machine chosen would have to have a large memory space, good colour graphics capabilities, support a range of standard language compilers, preferably offer some form of multi-tasking and job control, and be low cost. At the time the project started, only one machine fulfilled these requirements – the Sinclair QL, although the basic 128 K memory supplied had to be increased to 512 K for the purpose.

A consideration influencing the choice was the problem of where to hold the programs and data during operation. The conventional option of disc drives was expensive, whether as add-ons for those machines without them, or as a factor in the total costs of those with them built in. Data security problems were also posed with removable magnetic media, and in the interests of ensuring that data sets were consistent in that should a file of records be damaged, we could not contemplate the thought of the possible existence of several discs all purporting to hold the latest version of a particular file.

RAM discs offered a solution, when coupled with a mode of operation with the machines in use for long periods after initial loading with a master copy of the operating files. The RAM discs currently in use are extremely fast, capable of transferring information from storage to working memory at a rate of over 30 Mbytes/second and have the added advantage of being dynamic, occupying only little more than the space they need to hold their contents, rather than having to be formally formatted to a specific and inviolate size.

The Sinclair QL has had, in general, a rough ride from its critics; two particular areas singled out for attention being the microdrive tape systems, and overall reliability. The inadequacies of the microdrives are well documented, but we did not intend to make great use of them, and having purchased dual disc drives for developmental purposes the microdrives posed little problem. With regard to reliability, this has always seemed to be from our point of view a failure of quality control by the manufacturer as once any initial defect is corrected, little further trouble arises.

The basic physical set-up comprises the QL, a VDU of some description, and a serial cable connecting to the nearby Infaplug. The idle workstation runs a small Superbasic program inviting the user to log in and select from a small menu the mode of operation, and by implication, the files required for this. The program invokes the Kermit file transfer package to service this request, and then initiates the data-capture program, which finds its input on the RAM discs. On completion of operations, the updated records are written back to the RAM discs for conveyance back to the central file store by a further invocation of Kermit. The idle screen display is subsequently resumed.

The data-capture program is a product of a large proportion of the total time and effort spent on the project. Its function is to take as input one or more files corresponding to the lists of records previously mentioned, to allow the user to update or add to such records in a clear and rapid manner, while validating such amendments as strictly as possible within the limits defined for varying data fields, before allocating the records to the correct output files on the basis of their contents. It was decided that few conventional database capabilities were needed in the data-capture program, but the user would need some reminder of the numbers of records in the various categories, and a means of tracing records with a given entry in any one field, and these have been provided. Extensive use is made of the colour, graphics, and windowing facilities of the QL in the screen displays (Fig. 5.3).

To make life easier for the user of task-related screens, which present a combination of fields previously filled with those expected to be completed in the course of the specific task, the former are considered to be of use in the selection of entries for the latter. Each screen that the user sees may be considered as a page positioned in a two-dimensional matrix of such items. By a simple keying

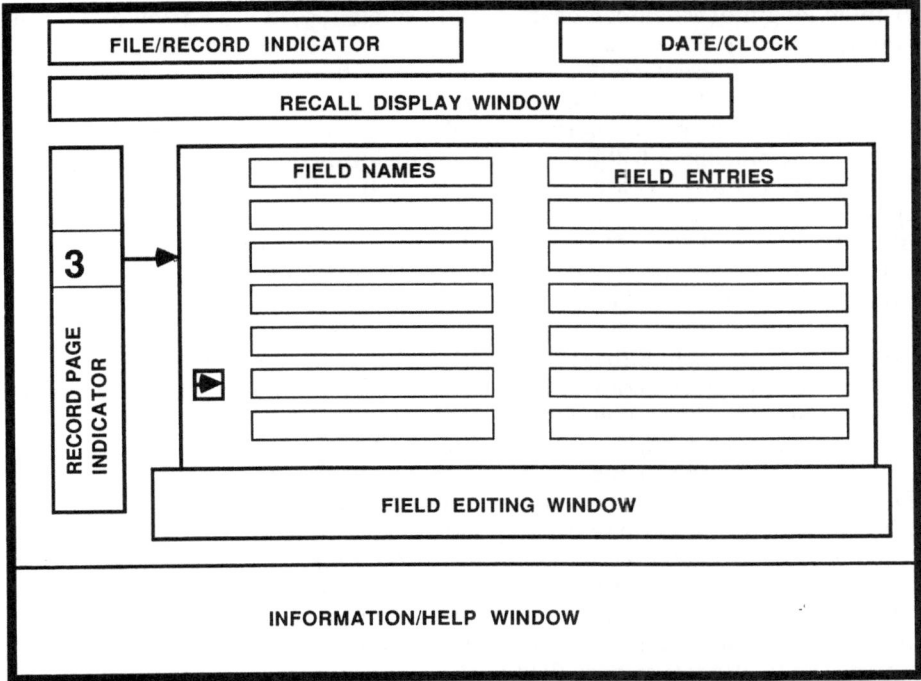

Fig. 5.3. Data-capture screen.

combination the user may cause the page above, below, left or right to be displayed, corresponding to the previous and next pages in the same patient record in the case of the first two movements, and the equivalent page of the two adjacent records in the latter pair.

Wrap-around capability is provided in all directions, and visual indication of the position of the current page within the imaginary matrix is given on a vertical basis by a graphical representation of a complete record card with the appropriate page highlighted and colour-coordinated with the background shade of the page in view. Indication of the lateral position of the current card is provided by a display of three figures such as 3/5/14. This particular example would show that there are fourteen records present in the workstation in total, and that the user is looking at the third record out of the five that have the same file number. The file type is also displayed here, colour-coded reinforcement of the reminder being provided by the strip colour of the indicator display reflecting that of the field names listed on the page in view.

Changing certain field entries for a particular record, the admission date, for example, whether by addition, amendment or deletion, causes changes to its file number, and possibly its file type. If such a change occurs, then the card record is moved in relation to the others present in the workstation to maintain the correct sort order, once the user leaves it for another one. The sort, also performed after record intake and before their output, is by ascending file number, which reflects implicitly ascending file types. Thus the user is presented with the records that have been selected, in the order corresponding to the main pattern of patient throughput.

All the field entries are held in the QL as ASCII strings with an arbitrary maximum length of seventeen characters. A single record is an array of a given number, currently 50, of such strings, space for each record being allocated dynamically. At present, with a 512 K memory, there is room for around 150 records, more than it is intended that a user should work with in any one session, and there is also always the option to add another 128 K of RAM to bring the QLs up to the maximum 640 K catered for. Obviously there are many fields that will never need the 17 character potential allotted to them. With these, and empty fields, to consider, it made sense to compress the record files for transmission around the network and storage on the hard disc, re-expanding them again on take-up by the QL. This is performed simply by adding a specified character as an end-of-field marker, ensuring of course that such a character can never be placed in a field by a user.

Although all the field entries consist of ASCII text, fewer than half of them are typed in through the conventional direct method of a line editing function. Those that are, may be termed the free-text fields, which have no restrictions on their input apart from length, a slightly restricted character set, and the removal of any more than one space character between two words.

Date fields are displayed in the dd/mm/yy format, but are presented for editing in the form of three corresponding figures, each of which may be incremented or decremented by use of the arrow keys. The routine keeps track of the legality of the changes made, adjusting one or more of the fields accordingly. An important addition is the ability to specify upper and lower limits to user manipulation, set by some relation to either the current day's date or the contents of another date field in the same record. It was the inability of commercial databases to offer such fine control over validation at the entry stage that ruled them unfit for our purposes, although those incorporating fourth-generation languages with provision for the insertion of lower level routines are now just beginning to offer such possibilities.

Many fields can be completed from a defined and limited number of possibilities, and where this number is five or less, the range is displayed in the editing window for the user to make a selection with the cursor keys. Besides permitting the user to complete such fields more rapidly, limiting free-text facilities is of great importance in the operation of the database construction from such entries.

Since many queries involve the selection of a subset of records from the total by virtue of the contents of one or more fields it is important that a single form of spelling, phrasing, or abbreviation will specify all the entries pertaining to that particular field or fields. It is also essential to maximise efficiency, notwithstanding any wild character or plain text retrieval capabilities a database may possess. Coding mechanisms are possible but it was decided that, for our purposes, the best solutions lay in the use of lists of standardised representations from which to make the valid choices for certain fields. The relational capabilities of Informix would theoretically permit the visual display screens to show the text form of a coded field from a look-up file, but the capacity of the Compaq Deskpro limited the use of this technique. The use of a relatively large number of joined files also reduces the speed at which queries can be answered, and the simplicity of construction of queries.

Defined data lists may be of great value in enabling standardisation, but there are two main practical problems. The first is to enable the user rapidly to convert his idea of the representation for a particular field into an actual entry in the computer-held record when there may be hundreds of possible choices. For such menu fields, the data-capture program opens a new window on the display when the user indicates the need to make an entry for that field, rather than use the double height character editing window that caters for the other types. A number of items are displayed vertically within the window, together with a bar that may be moved to rest across each item, in response to the cursor keys. The window features wrap-around scrolling of the item list, should there be more items than can be displayed at once in the window. If there are a great many items this would defeat the object of the exercise, so a hierarchical structure involving higher level menus is imposed upon the raw list to enable users to step through quickly to their area of choice. Pressing the return key selects the item currently under the bar, which may either be the actual entry for the field, or an indicator of the next menu in the hierarchy to be presented. Both types may simultaneously exist in the same presented menu.

The second problem is the one of construction of the lists, and hence of which choices to present to the user. Taking the example of diagnoses, although one aim of the project is to provide the RHA with the WHO codes, it is clearly impossible to hold every coded diagnosis in the menu system. So a selection was made consisting only of those diagnoses likely to be encountered at least once during an average year's workload in the Department. It is interesting to note that although the WHO codings may be over-specific for the purposes of surgical audit, in a number of cases the reverse applies and we classify several separate diagnoses which WHO codes with one entry. Having imposed such restrictions solves one problem to create another i.e. recording those cases not listed in the menus.

The hierarchical menu mechanism, besides offering the selected options, also provides some additional features. There is the ability to go back from lower menu levels to the previous menu, together with the feature of free text entry of a diagnosis, when the user considers there is no suitable corresponding keyword in the menu. Such field entries are prefaced with an asterisk for easy subsequent extraction from the database, with a view to considering their inclusion in the normal menu should numbers warrant. Conversely it is also possible to monitor the frequency of use of the formal menu entries in order to remove unnecessary ones.

A final field type is that of the hidden field which, as its name implies, is not presented to the user, although it forms part of an individual patient record. Neither can the user write to such a field directly, although the other changes made to the record may cause alterations to the field contents. Such fields are used internally by the data-capture program, recording for example the file number and type, or on an external basis to see when, and/or by whom, a particular record was last altered.

Fields do not necessarily start empty when a new record is begun. Several fields can be completed by default, either on an overall basis by virtue of the probabilities involved in a limited range of choices, or by implication upon the entry of other items. An example of this is provisional entry of an operation date two days subsequent to the admission date when this field is filled. Doing this leaves the user free to bypass the machine-made entries in the majority of cases, hence saving time, but leaving the option of alteration should it be required.

One other special case is where a field can only be filled or edited by the user after entering a previous field. This would seem on the face of it to be an inconvenience, but in fact provides a means of correctly coordinating the entries in two or more fields. In the single example of this currently utilised, no operations menu can be obtained without the immediately previous selection of a diagnosis from the menus pertaining to that field. In this manner it is ensured that only the operations thought appropriate with that choice of diagnosis are offered as the menu for that field, together with the standing options of "no operation" or recourse to free text as mentioned previously.

There are two consequences of the provision of user assistance in the form of menu systems. The first is that if the contents of the menu lists are variable over time, as they are to permit maximum adaptability, no reference to the absolute position of a particular item in relation to its parent menu should be carried within a record. This has the practical effect that any alteration to the contents of a menu field can only be made by starting at the top of the hierarchy tree and working through again. As there are at most four levels in any one menu system this is thought a small price to pay for the provision of updatable selections obviating both validation problems and the chore of text entry.

The second is that to avoid wholesale recompilation of the program for each minor change to a menu list, such items should be held outside the program code. This is a manifestation of the fundamental philosophy underlying the construction of the data-capture program, which is to implement a bare framework capable of self-configuration from externally held variable items, ranging from the high level of field menu lists, through the positioning of fields on pages, down to the detail of window sizings and colour schemes. Again a price is paid in that time is taken when the program starts up, as it loads its run time variables into the various internal arrays set up to hold them, but this is offset to some extent by the reduction in compilation, and hence overall development, time. Loading takes place within one minute as all the necessary format and menu files are held on the RAM discs and, being in ASCII form, it is easy to edit them and transmit them across the network.

There are a number of other features of the displays presented to the user that are worth noting. A real time clock display mounted by a small low-priority machine-code program operates continuously and concurrently with all the other software in the QL, to provide a quick reference for users and an indication of the correct function of the machine as it updates roughly every second, subject to other job loads. As the internal clock/calendar is frequently used in setting limits and defaults for date field entry, its continual display will alert the user should it be inaccurate for any reason.

It is also useful while looking at one page of a record to be able to review the contents of fields on other pages, without having to change to those pages. This facility is provided by means of a recall window, through which the contents of one field at a time may be called up in sequence. The field is set by default to display the family name of the patient in the current record, but any alteration will hold, displaying the contents of the chosen field as the user moves from page to page or record to record.

A further window at the bottom of the display provides a quick help reference to the actions of various keys for the task in hand. One of these will call up a more comprehensive help screen introducing the concepts of the program and detailing all the possible actions. The program is driven at all times by single and combined key presses. No command lines or phrases are necessary. It is possible to add a new record, and to move directly to the first and last records. The most involved routine is one to find and display the first record encountered to the right of the current one with an entry in a chosen field corresponding to a requested search string. There is nothing in the program to inhibit the addition of further functions, should they be defined, for example to place a restricted amount of information on several patients simultaneously on the same screen.

Data security is an obvious consideration when handling patients' personal medical records. A large proportion of potential misuse has been negated by avoiding any storage of these on transportable magnetic media, and by the construction of programs blocking direct user interface to the operating system of the workstations. Although some form of protection is given by the need for password access, a factor encountered in having medical staff providing some of the data entry is that they may be called away from the workstation urgently to attend a patient. Although the workstations are not placed in designated public thoroughfares, it is obviously undesirable that data should remain displayed in the absence of the operator. A timeout is therefore operated, in that if a keypress has not been detected for an externally defined length of time, the screen display is cleared and the password needs to be re-entered before the session can be continued.

Particularly important in a system based on single exclusive use of served files, is that such files are returned to the server within a reasonable time interval to permit others to have access to them. Hence a second overall timeout operates in that as the data-capture program starts, the internal clock is read and the user informed of the time by which transactions should be completed. Attempts to exceed this time result in the program shutting itself down, in order to return files to the server.

As the data-capture program starts it may be the case that the user has not obtained all the files requested for the indicated operating mode, and has to make do with those that have been obtained, or log on at a later time. This is the most visible manifestation of the decision not to use a true multi-user system, but is essential to avoid the possibility of the coexistence of differing versions of the same file. By the use of the timeout feature, and the fact that the main list divisions are themselves divided in a number of ways to form individual files (Fig. 5.4), such disappointments can be kept to a minimum. The practical working patterns of staff and their needs for information at certain times at predictable locations also tends to mitigate the effects of the theoretical disadvantages inherent in such file-locking.

The workstations are intended to be left in operation for as long a period as possible, thus conserving the contents of the RAM discs. A cold start-up involves 1–2 minutes for loading the three main programs and the format files, setting the clock/calendar and running a small test on the correct functioning of the pathways to the file server. At one time it was hoped to use an EPROM board to hold the main routines, but the total size of the code involved would mean the use of an extension board capable of supporting a number of EPROM devices, and a programming device capable of blowing one file across more than one of them, neither of which are readily available at present.

LIST TYPE

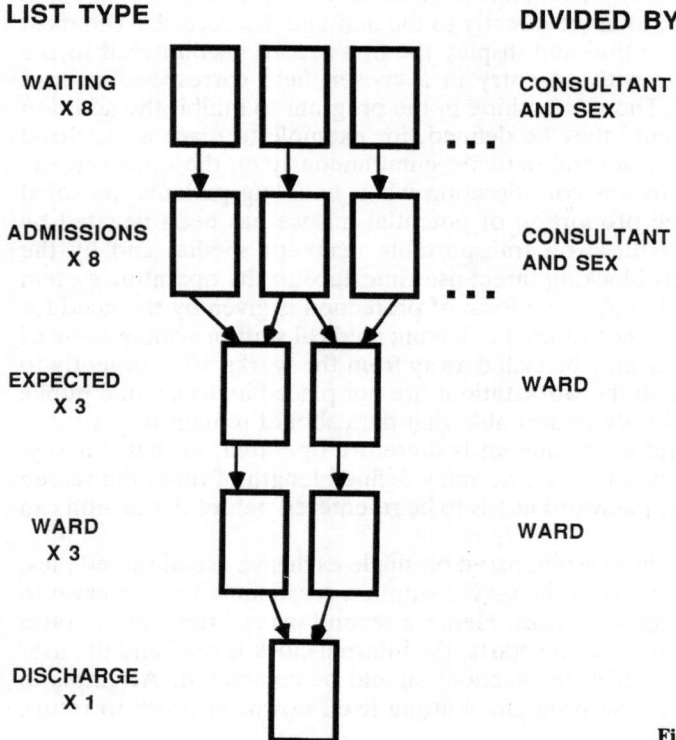

DIVIDED BY

WAITING
X 8

CONSULTANT
AND SEX

ADMISSIONS
X 8

CONSULTANT
AND SEX

EXPECTED
X 3

WARD

WARD
X 3

WARD

DISCHARGE
X 1

Fig. 5.4. Patient record files.

The Current State

At the time of writing the Informix database has been in use for 6 months, data have been collected by the house officers on paper forms approximating to the data capture screens. Comparison of database statistics with those from other sources has confirmed that such a method of collection is prone to error and omission, as well as suffering from time lags as the task is given a low priority. At the same time, the powerful potential of this new tool has been recognised and utilised, within the Department, and also by the RHA.

The installation of the network cabling in the hospital is complete and the system has been tested within the confines of a single room. After a trial period it is hoped to extend the system to the secretarial staff for patient administration. We hope to place similar systems, subject to operating experience in other hospitals associated with the Department, to widen the scope of the audit database.

References

1 Dudly HAF (1974) Necessity for surgical audit. Br Med J 1: 275–277
2 Gough MH et al. (1980) An annual assessment of the work and performance of a surgical firm in a regional teaching hospital. Br Med J 2: 913–915.
3 Korner E (1982) Steering group on health services information. HMSO, London
4 Griffiths R (1983) Griffiths Report. HMSO, London

Commercial Information

5 Xenix, Informix: Logica (UK) Ltd, 64 Newman Street, London W1A 4SE, UK
6 Compaq Deskpro: Compaq Computer Corporation, Houston, Texas 77070, USA
7 Infaplug: Infa Communications Ltd, Bath Place, Taunton TA1 4EP, UK
8 Kermit Protocol Manual (5th edition 1984): Columbia University, New York, NY, USA

6 Computerised Analysis of Vascular Laboratory Data

P.D. Coleridge Smith and J.H. Scurr

Introduction

In the vascular laboratory at the Middlesex Hospital we perform many tests of arterial and venous function. The tests of arterial function use Doppler ultrasound and involve recording the velocity waveforms and ankle systolic pressures. Investigations of venous function include photoplethysmography and foot volumetry, tests for reflux and a strain gauge test for venous outflow. We also have facilities for measuring the pressure in the dorsal foot vein during ambulation as an assessment of venous function and reflux. Originally all these tests were performed with the aid of dual-channel chart recorders which produced one trace for each lower limb. This inevitably produced large amounts of data, many of which were not used in evaluating the patient and required the application of ruler and calculator to determine the parameters we wished to know. The process of examining the recorded traces and producing the final report was therefore very time-consuming and significantly reduced the numbers of patients that could be investigated by one person. It was with these problems in mind that we turned to the computer for help with the tasks of the vascular laboratory.

Investigations and Parameters

In the investigation of arterial disease, examination of the Doppler ultrasound traces forms a useful screening test of vascular function. In these investigations a probe containing two ultrasonic transducers is placed over the artery to be examined. A transmitter transducer emits ultrasonic energy at 5–8 MHz. This is reflected from many structures in the tissues, but moving blood is the component that will impart a Doppler shift on the impinging signal. The received signal is amplified and converted to voltage signal at the output of the Doppler machine which represents the instantaneous Doppler shift, and hence velocity of the blood in the artery. This is usually recorded on a chart recorder to obtain a permanent record. The traces themselves are of most use to the clinician: although attempts have been made to derive numerical values from the traces, these have generally been of no greater use than the traces alone.

In venous disease the photoplethysmograph (PPG) is used in our laboratory as a test of venous reflux. This simple device has a transducer head containing a light emitting diode operating at about 800nm and a phototransistor to detect the returning light. The transducer is attached to the skin of the lower limb by means of adhesive tape. The light reaching the phototransistor must traverse the skin and its intensity is therefore dependent on the transmission of light by the skin. At the wavelength chosen, the skin becomes less transmissive to the light as the

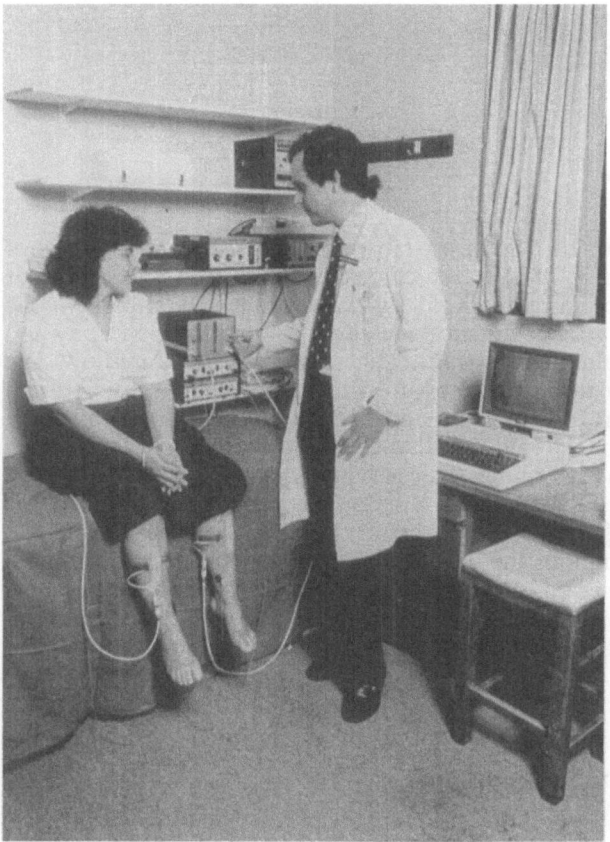

Fig. 6.1. Photoplethysmography refilling test for venous reflux. The patient performs ten dorsiflexions of the ankle to empty the calf veins.

small veins and capillaries fill. The state of fullness or emptiness of these vessels can therefore be deduced in a semi-quantitative way. The most useful parameter that may be extracted is the time taken for venous refilling following a standard exercise. In this test the patient sits or stands and then performs ten dorsiflexions of the ankle (Fig. 6.1). This causes contraction of the calf muscles which empties the calf veins. The time taken for the veins to refill is an index of the amount of reverse flow down veins in which the valves have failed. In normal subjects no reverse flow occurs and refilling is attributable to arterial inflow to the leg. In patients with varicose veins or venous ulcers much more rapid refilling occurs, due to reverse flow along the damaged veins. In providing a report of the examination of a particular patient the trace is useful to assist the clinician in determining whether there was any artificial alteration in the refilling time, which may not be apparent if the refilling time alone were quoted.

We also use a Thulesius foot volumeter to determine refilling time as an adjunct to PPG, particularly in research applications (Fig. 6.2). This device measures the change in foot volume following a standard exercise by detecting changes in the level of water in a foot bath. Similar data to those from the

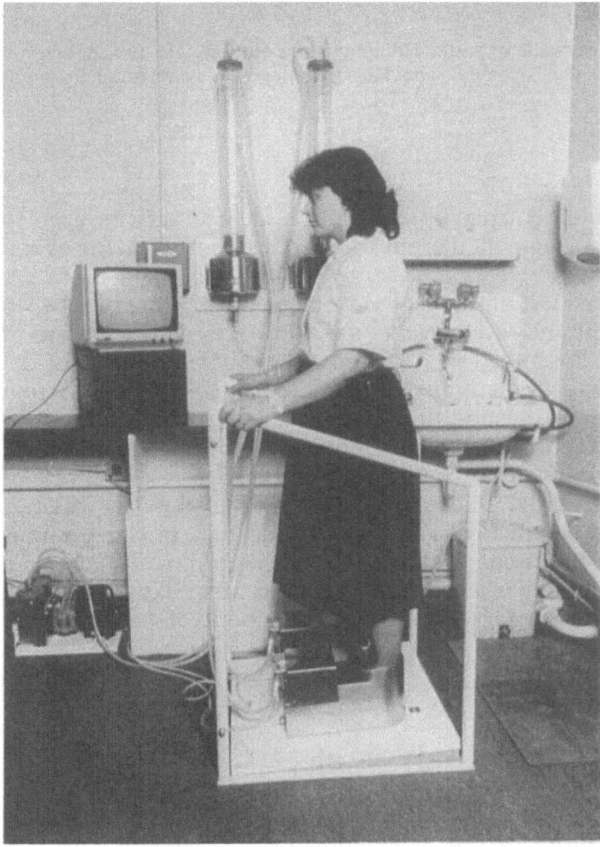

Fig. 6.2. A Thulesius foot volumeter in use. The patient performs 10 knee-bends to empty the calf veins and then stands at rest while refilling of the foot venous compartment takes place.

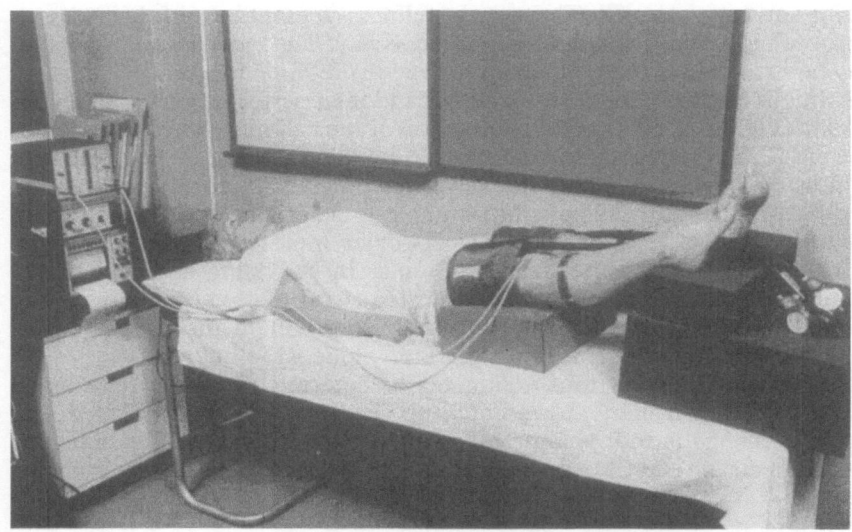

Fig. 6.3. Measurement of venous capacitance and maximum venous outflow. The patient lies still while the thigh cuff is inflated and then deflated. The calf circumference is measured by strain gauges.

photoplethysmograph are obtained, but in addition the device may be used to determine the volume of blood expelled from the venous compartment of the foot during exercise.

In the assessment of obstruction of the major veins from the lower limbs we use strain gauges to determine the rate of venous outflow following a period of venous occlusion with a cuff. With the feet elevated 25 cm above the level of the heart, cuffs are placed around both thighs and inflated to 55 mm Hg. Strain gauges composed of mercury in silastic tubing are wrapped around the legs to measure changes in circumference. After two minutes of compression, which occludes all major veins in the lower limbs, the cuffs are deflated and the rate of outflow measured during the initial 1 second of emptying (Fig. 6.3). This test allows both the ability of the venous compartment to increase in size (venous capacitance) as well as the venous outflow to be determined. It is an investigation useful for determining whether deep vein thrombosis is present in a patient presenting with a swollen leg and in the assessment of patients with long-standing venous ulcers.

Recording, Reporting and Analysis of Data

Various tasks can be recognised in the production of a vascular laboratory report. The first is the recording of data for subsequent analysis. This usually involves inspecting the traces obtained while continuously monitoring the output of the transducer amplifier concerned. Much of the trace will be rejected while adjustments are made and these data therefore need not be recorded at all. The display of a graph on large axes with clearly coloured lines is useful for ease of recognising the trace from each transducer. The ability to add comments to the recorded data which will appear on the final report is also useful. The recording of the data required is the next stage. This will be in a form which can be analysed by a computer in the generation of any subsequent report. The output from ordinary chart recorders cannot be read directly by computers, and is therefore unsuitable for this application. Magnetic recording techniques are necessary as data can then be read directly into the computer for further processing. The analyses themselves may be far more complex and rigorous if a computer is used. For example, performing a least squares fit to obtain the best correlation line for a set of data would be slow if performed by hand but takes the computer a few seconds, allowing a more complete analysis to be obtained without any extra effort by the investigator. Finally, a report should be generated. It is extremely tedious to have to cut up pieces of chart recorder paper and attach them to a report form and then annotate the form appropriately. Computers may generate reports in various ways to include graphs, charts, traces as well as numerical data without the need for a glue-pot!

Connecting the Laboratory Equipment to a Computer

The output from the transducer amplifiers is intended to be attached to a chart recorder and ranges between ±2–3 volts depending on the equipment and the tests performed. Computers unfortunately do not understand the continuously varying parameters of the real world and must assign numerical values to any such input. The actual piece of hardware that achieves this is an analogue to digital convertor (A/D). In our system we used a device capable of reading eight different inputs and representing voltages over the range of 0–2.5 volts by a number between 0 and 255. A preamplifier system was added (PMS Instruments Ltd, Maidenhead, Berks) which converts all transducer amplifier outputs to this voltage range and prevents damaging voltages being applied to the A/D. The computer system we use is the BBC microcomputer (Acorn Computer, Cambridge) interfaced to the A/D convertor. This computer system was already available in our department and several computers are connected together using a network, sharing expensive devices such as a letter-quality printer and hard disc drive. All users of the system keep their programs on the hard disc, although floppy discs are also in use at several of the computers for additional storage of data.

Software

Programs were written in BBC BASIC, a high level language which is both easy to write and exploits the full capabilities of the computer. Some sections of the software had to work very quickly and were written in 6502 assembly language which was converted to machine code by the BASIC assembler program. This is the lowest level language of the system and is somewhat unforgiving of programming errors, though it offers the fastest means of achieving most tasks. Various philosophies were agreed upon in writing these programs:

1. The need for simple operation means that menus of options should be presented to the user. The possible functions of the programs can be clearly displayed at any particular point when a decision is to be made by the user.

2. Where graphical data are to be presented it should be possible first to run the program continuously while adjustments are made to the transducers and then to select only the part of the trace that contains useful data.

3. It should be possible to add comments to traces by typing at the keyboard when the trace is recorded, rather than committing details to memory for later transfer to paper.

4. The analysis of data should be automatic so that the user is not required to participate in analysis decisions.

We decided that it was desirable to produce graphical representation of data on the final report. One solution to this has been to use a plotter to draw the graphs. This has the advantage of producing high quality reports, but text and reports with many lines are slow to generate. It remains satisfactory for some reports, but most are produced on a dot-matrix printer. The latter has the advantage that it can print relatively quickly, but produces a lower quality report. The graphics have proved satisfactory for most purposes and readily readable graphs are produced.

Doppler Ultrasound Programs

In these programs we decided that it was appropriate to record the trace from each of four arteries in either lower limb along with patient data (name, number, etc) and ankle pressures before and after exercise. A complete patient record would be a set of eight traces plus the patient data. We decided to hold the patient data on a floppy disc and up to 31 sets of traces are stored on each side of a disc.

The Doppler traces are displayed on the computer screen, being drawn from left to right, then re-starting at the left of the screen and replacing the previous trace when the right edge is reached (Fig. 6.4). This means that the input from the Doppler probe can be continuously displayed until a satisfactory trace is obtained. The user signals to the computer that he is satisfied with the trace by pressing a foot-switch or a key on the computer keyboard. The computer checks whether either of these have been pressed after each new point is plotted on the screen, that is, at a rate of 100 times per second. Once the switch is pressed the computer stops plotting the data from the Doppler input. It clears the screen and re-draws the last 320 points, starting at the left edge of the screen. The design of the program is such that these data are always available, so it is not necessary to wait until the screen edge is reached before pressing the switch. The trace displayed is therefore the last 3.2 seconds of the recording. This fills the screen and will eventually occupy about 3.2 inches of paper in the final report giving a trace speed of 1 inch per second. A further press of the foot-switch transfers this record to the floppy disc as a permanent record in that patient's file. The

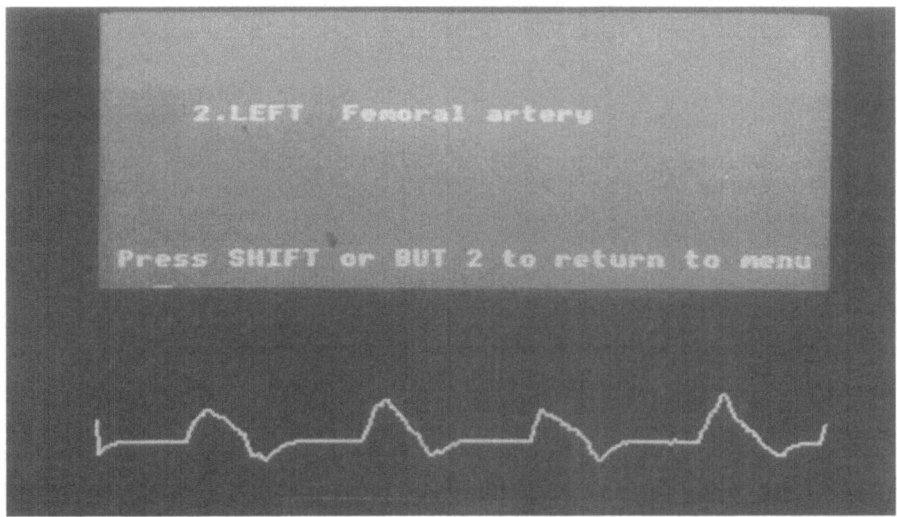

Fig. 6.4. A Doppler ultrasound trace displayed on the computer screen.

Table 6.1. Order of vessels expected by the Doppler ultrasound program

Right femoral artery
Left femoral artery
Right popliteal artery
Left popliteal artery
Right dorsalis pedis artery
Left dorsalis pedis artery
Right posterior tibial artery
Left posterior tibial artery

computer then displays a menu offering the next trace to be recorded. It goes through the vessels to be examined in a logical order (Table 6.1). If an error is made a second foot-switch allows a previously recorded trace to be over-written by a new trace. Traces already recorded must be specifically over-written by the use of the second foot-switch, a feature which prevents the accidental erasure of data. Finally a menu (Table 6.2) is available for the recording of patient data, including ankle systolic pressures before and after exercise.

After a session in which one or several patients' sets of data have been recorded, the report-generating program is selected from the menu. Two versions of this are currently in use. The first uses a plotter to draw a multi-colour report. The second prints reports using an ordinary dot-matrix printer, in which the colours are restricted to black on white! Examples of each are shown in Figs 6.5 and 6.6. Although coloured reports are more aesthetic the paper must be hand-loaded and thus only one report can be generated at once. The program for the printer reads the floppy disc and displays the names of files containing Doppler traces. It offers the option of printing any file or combination of files, including all of them. Each takes 2–3 minutes to print so that a full disc of 31

Table 6.2. Patient details and data collected by the Doppler ultrasound program

Last name
First name
Hospital number
Age
Sex
Department
Comment
Brachial pressure
Right ankle systolic pressure
Left ankle systolic pressure
Post-exercise brachial pressure
Post-exercise right ASP
Post-exercise left ASP

traces would take over an hour to complete. In this case the computer could be left to finish its task at the end of the day.

As can be seen the final report contains patient data and ankle pressures. In this case the only calculations necessary have been the generation of the ankle – brachial systolic indices.

Software Problems and Techniques

In writing this part of the software it was necessary continuously to display the data from the Doppler chart recorder output and store the trace for future use. Initially it was thought to be desirable that the trace scroll across the screen horizontally to simulate the usual chart recorder used for these machines. Unfortunately, this is not easy to achieve. The memory used to generate the display in mode 1 on the BBC microcomputer screen is 20 Kbytes. Only half of this is actually used for the trace, the remainder being assigned to text. In order to achieve a smooth scroll horizontally it would be necessary to move this trace one pixel to the left fast enough to keep up with the correct display speed. Since the horizontal resolution of the screen is 320 pixels, and represents 3.2 seconds, this would have meant scrolling the screen every 10 milliseconds or at 100 Hz. The rate of moving memory would be $100 \times 10\,K = 1$ Mbyte/second. The microprocessor in the BBC microcomputer cannot achieve such speeds without hardware assistance, and so another solution was found.

We decided that the display could remain still, but would be continuously updated with current data which would over-write the previous trace. Initially the screen is cleared and the trace commences at the left-hand edge. On reaching the right edge of the screen the trace re-commences on the left replacing the previous trace. In order to achieve this effect some means of erasing the existing trace was necessary. Initially we tried to erase all pixels in the column immediately ahead of the writing position, but this proved to be too slow. A more complex algorithm was devised. A block of memory 320 bytes long (one for each horizontal screen position) is reserved to save data read from the A/D convertor. On first displaying the trace the data are plotted to the screen as well as being saved in memory. During the second and subsequent scans of the screen the memory contains the coordinates of the line plotted on the previous scan.

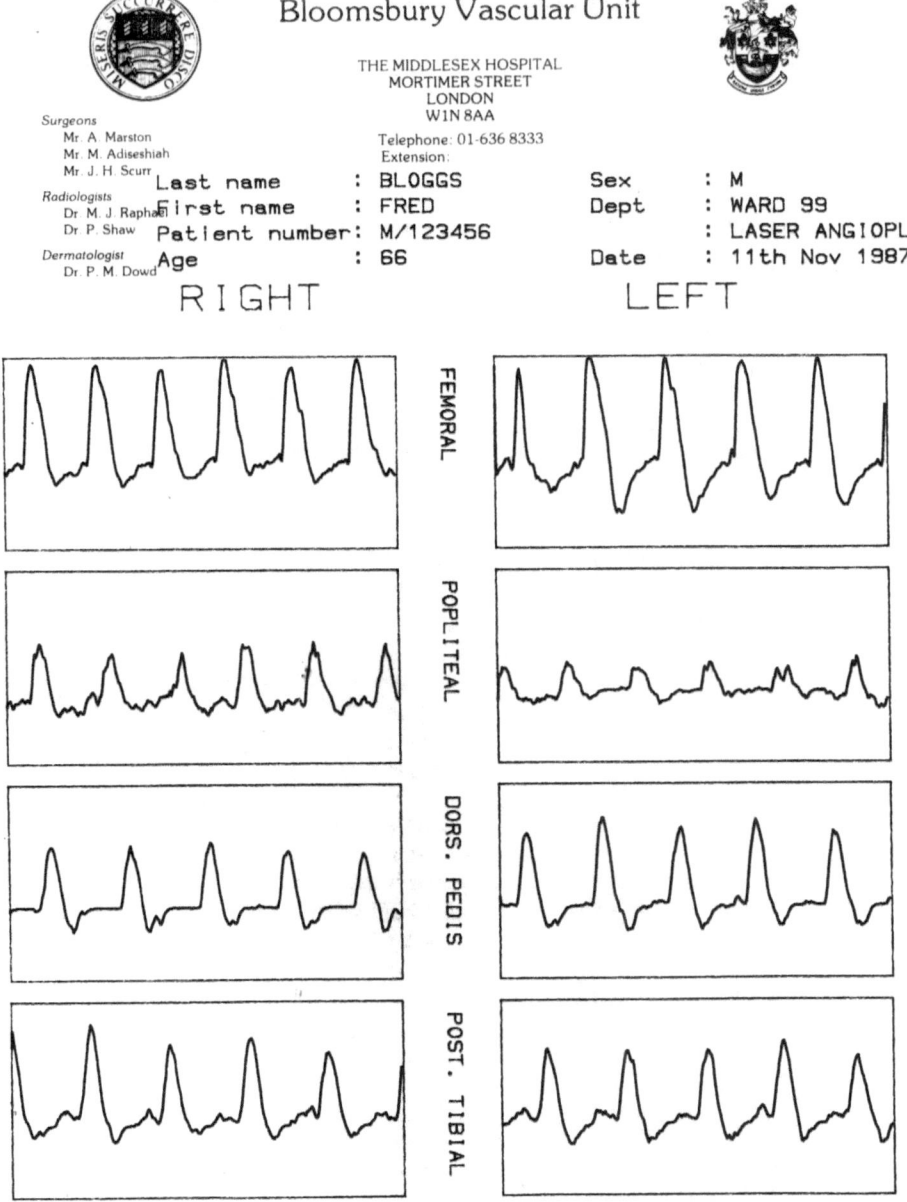

Fig. 6.5. Report from the Doppler ultrasound program produced with the plotter.

Bloomsbury Vascular Unit
Vascular Laboratory

Last name   : BLOGGS   Sex   : M
First name   : FRED   Dept : WARD 99
Patient number: M/123456   : LASER ANGIOPL.
Age   : 66

Date of examination: 11th Nov 1987

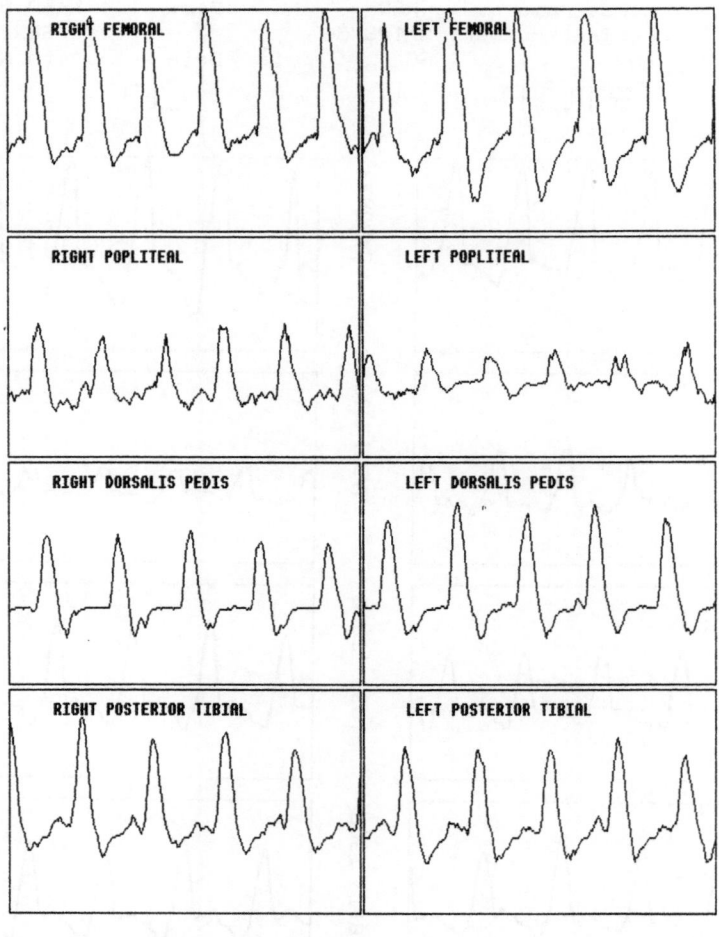

Resting ankle syst press.....:   125   125
Index.........................:   1.00   1.00
Post exercise ASP.............:   145   145
Index.........................:   1.04   1.04

Fig. 6.6. Report from the Doppler ultrasound program produced on a matrix printer.

This is then re-plotted in the background colour to remove the line. The new data are then put into the memory area and plotted in the foreground colour. This technique means that only those pixels which were set to the foreground colour are addressed during the erasing process, and is much faster than the previous technique.

The requirement of the screen display algorithm to use a memory buffer to hold the incoming data is not disadvantageous since these data must be held in memory before transfer to disc. The machine will always have access to the previous 320 bytes (3.2 seconds) of data read from the A/D, and so recording of data is facilitated by the screen handling technique. The start of the trace may not correspond with the start of the memory buffer, but it is not necessary to shuffle the data about. All the machine must remember is the start location of the data in memory. It plots these data at the left edge of the screen and then moves on sequentially through the remaining data, moving back to the beginning of the memory buffer on reaching the end and continuing until all points have been plotted. This is done by both the input software and the report-generating software. The start position of the data is held in the 2 bytes which follow the data area in the memory buffer. These are written to when the person using the equipment presses the space bar or the foot-switch to indicate satisfaction with the recorded data. This allows the trace to be re-drawn with the most recent point at the right edge of the screen. The data are then saved on disc keeping both trace and starting point information together as a 322 byte record in a patient's file.

Data are transferred to disc using an operating system call (called OSGBPB) available only from machine code. This transfers a block of data from memory to disc by a single call to the subroutine. Memory may be restored from disc by using the same routine. This operating system routine is used to store records for each patient in a single file. It is also used to put the data back into memory so that they may be displayed. Eight of the records contain the Doppler traces, the remainder are used to hold patient information (name, number, address). The latter is put in the memory buffer area by a further operating system command which puts characters into a user defined place in memory and allows simple editing. For simplicity, the memory buffer area was used so that it could be saved to disc using the same part of the program that is used to save the Doppler traces. Since it is always the first record in the file there is no confusion about which record holds trace and which holds patient information.

The reports generated by this part of the software principally contain the trace data, although patient data including ankle blood pressures is also included. We intended that all reports would be plotted using an XY plotter, but it subsequently became apparent that such devices were too large for portable use and versions of the program which produce a report on a matrix printer were devised.

The DXY–880 plotter (Roland DG, Great West Road, Brentford, Middlesex) uses a graphics language compatible with the Hewlett-Packard Graphics Language (HPGL). The command structure is fairly simple and includes a number of advanced commands which facilitate the generation of reports. For plotting traces the plot absolute (PA) and plot relative commands are used. These require the use of parameters in plotter coordinates (of 0.2 mm), for example:

PA 200 100;

would move the pen to x position 200, y position 100. The pen contact is controlled by pen-up (PU) and pen-down (PD) commands. It is easily envisaged how a graph may be plotted using the commands. The data for the patient traces is read from disc and multiplied by a scaling factor to make it the right size for the plotter. A PA command is then constructed (using BASIC) and sent to the plotter using the serial interface. This is repeated for each point in the record. All eight traces are drawn in this way for each file. The rectangles around the traces are drawn using the Edge Rectangle Absolute command (EA), which requires only the coordinates of the diagonal of the rectangle. Annotation is added using the internal character set of the plotter, which as can be seen in Fig. 6.7 may be reproduced in any size or orientation. Various colours for the different parts of the report are drawn by different pens. These are selected under software control using the select pen (SP) command. Up to eight different colours may be used with this particular type of plotter.

Generating the reports with a matrix printer is straightforward. The traces are drawn on the screen in the highest resolution mode (mode 0) giving 640 pixels horizontally by 256 vertically. Four traces at a time are accommodated on the screen and are plotted from the patient data on disc using the standard BBC BASIC plot commands. The software then calls a screen dump routine which copies the screen contents to the printer. The process is repeated for the next set

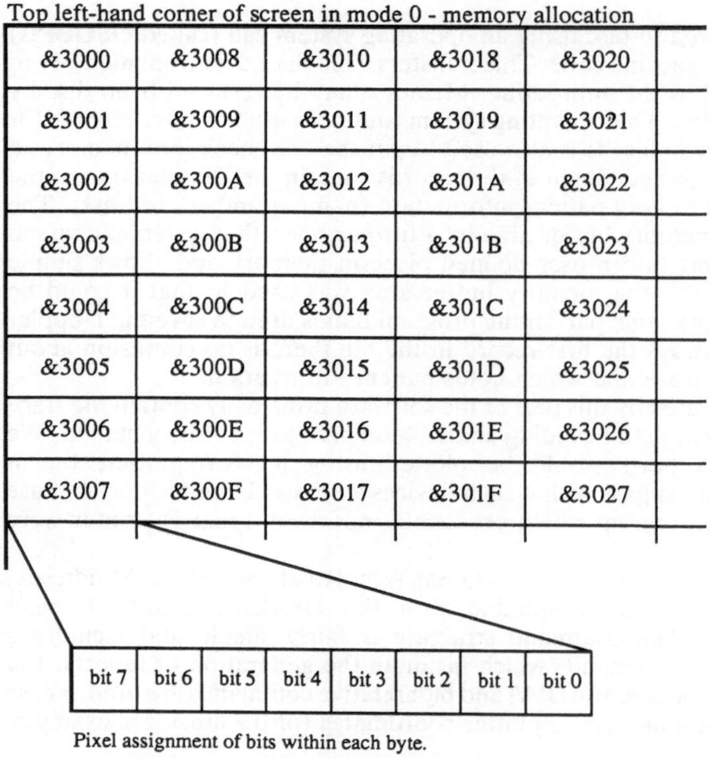

Top left-hand corner of screen in mode 0 - memory allocation

&3000	&3008	&3010	&3018	&3020	
&3001	&3009	&3011	&3019	&3021	
&3002	&300A	&3012	&301A	&3022	
&3003	&300B	&3013	&301B	&3023	
&3004	&300C	&3014	&301C	&3024	
&3005	&300D	&3015	&301D	&3025	
&3006	&300E	&3016	&301E	&3026	
&3007	&300F	&3017	&301F	&3027	

| bit 7 | bit 6 | bit 5 | bit 4 | bit 3 | bit 2 | bit 1 | bit 0 |

Pixel assignment of bits within each byte.

Fig. 6.7.   Screen memory arrangement in screen mode 0 on a BBC microcomputer.

of four traces. The header and patient data are added using conventional printer facilities. The screen dump used initially was one which employed the graphics cursor to read the pixel values at every point on the screen from which suitable data for the printer could be generated. This has the advantage that it works in all screen modes, including later models of the computer, without modification. But, even in machine code, it is rather slow. This became very apparent when it was used with a fast matrix printer. A modified version was written which reads screen memory directly and converts this to printer compatible format.

In screen mode 0 this is uncomplicated. Following a screen clear command, the top left-hand corner of the screen is represented by memory location &3000 (3000 hexadecimal). The first eight pixels in the top row correspond to bits 7 to 0 of this byte (Fig. 6.7). The first eight pixels in the next row are from byte &3001, and so on until location &3007. The next byte (&3008) is then on the first row again. This pattern continues throughout the screen. The printer requires pin patterns which correspond to the printer pins (Fig. 6.8). These are arranged vertically above each other, so that the first byte sent to the printer will have bit 7 of location &3000 as bit 7, bit 7 of location &3001 as bit 6 and so on until byte &3007. This is then sent to the printer, which has been warned to expect graphics data by an appropriate escape sequence. Following this all the bits 6 are sent, then bits 5 until bit 0 is reached. The next set of eight bytes is then sent.

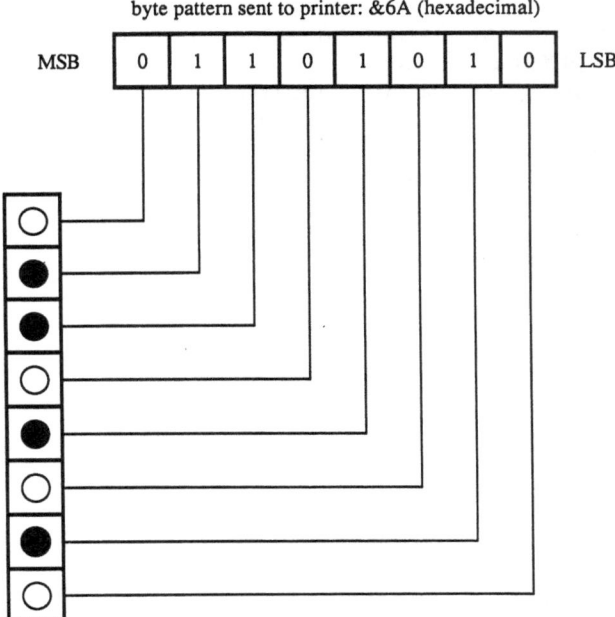

byte pattern sent to printer: &6A (hexadecimal)

dot pattern printed (single vertical row of dots)

Fig. 6.8. Pin patterns on a dot matrix printer and their relationship to data sent to be printed in graphics mode.

The process is then continued until the end of the line is reached. The printer is instructed to perform a line feed and re-start the process until all 32 lines have been dumped. This un-official dump works twice as fast as the fully compatible version on most printers.

The ability to print reports on continuous stationery allowed us to write an addition to the software to permit the generation of reports on all files on a disc. An operating system machine code command is used to read the names of all files on a disc; those which are of the correct length are assumed to contain Doppler traces. The names of all Doppler files on a disc are entered into an array and displayed on the screen with a number against each. The user may type a number which highlights the corresponding filename in inverse video. As many filenames as required may be selected. The selected ones are remembered by the program by setting a second element in the array to 1, instead of its initial null value. The computer then works its way through the array of filenames printing any that have a 1 in the second element of the array. The reports, although less elegant than those of the plotter, have high resolution and are adequate for most purposes.

Plethysmography Programs

All the plethysmography programs are based on a single original program written for photoplethysmography traces. The data are displayed in a similar way but the analyses are different. Again programs are selected from a menu (Fig. 6.9), allowing easy program selection.

The first option in the menu Run chart turns the computer screen into a chart recorder display (Fig. 6.10). On the vertical axis is the output voltage from the transducer amplifiers and time is on the horizontal axis. The program was originally developed to draw four inputs at once. The screen colours allow identification of each trace from the key. As can be seen, the traces progress from left to right of the screen and are more easily read than from a chart recorder where progress is usually from bottom to top of the page. The screen

```
    1......Run chart

    2......Data analysis

    3......See current data

    4......Save/Load data on disc

    5......Calibrate system

    6......Exit
```

Fig. 6.9. First menu of the plethysmography programs.

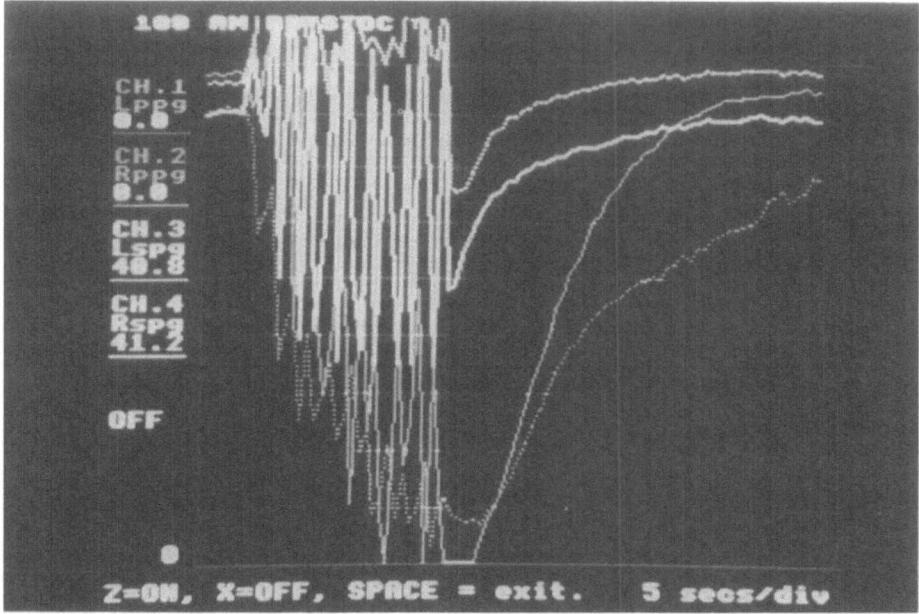

Fig. 6.10. An example of the screen display during data input from the photoplethysmography and strain gauge transducers from a venous refilling time test.

will only display 35 seconds of the recording at once but this disadvantage is overcome by scrolling the "paper" within the axes to the left when the traces reach the right edge of the screen. In this way the traces may be displayed continuously without time limit while equipment is adjusted. Data are transferred continuously to the computer memory when recording mode is switched on. This is done by pressing the Z key on the computer keyboard. A vertical white cursor appears on the screen to mark the start of the recording and each channel is then read to the computer memory every 400 milliseconds. Limitations in computer memory restrict the recording to 100 seconds in length, but this has been found to be long enough for most purposes. Recording may be terminated at any time by pressing the X key, limiting the length of the recorded trace. The menu may now be regained by pressing the space bar and various options are available. The trace may be reviewed with option 3 (Fig. 6.9), or transferred to disc using option 4. There is provision for recording patient data with each patient's file, which is capable of holding up to sixteen sets (of four) traces. In addition a typed comment may be appended to each trace for future identification, and will appear on the final report. A facility is also provided to include a calibration level with the recorded data from each channel. This is useful for the strain gauge and foot volumeter programs where it is essential to insert a 1 % or 5 ml calibration signal respectively. This permits future quantitative analysis of the traces.

THE MIDDLESEX HOSPITAL
Vascular Laboratory
Venous Assessment

Name: Fred Jones   Number: 123456   Ward: Charles Bell   Date: 1/4/86

PPG   Record number 0   Normal lower limbs

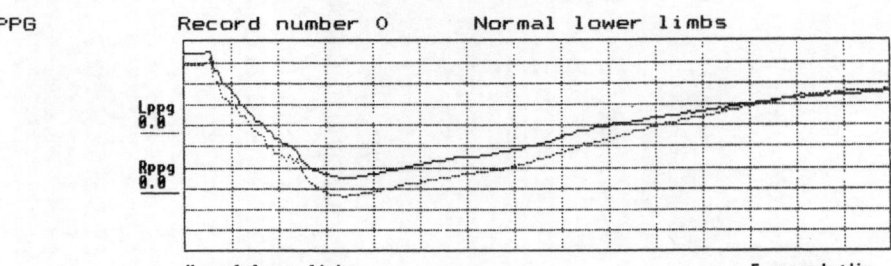

    Normal lower limbs   5 seconds/div

Photoplethysmography RIGHT LEFT
Refilling time (secs) 134.4 169.3

PPG   Record number 1   Bilateral varicose veins

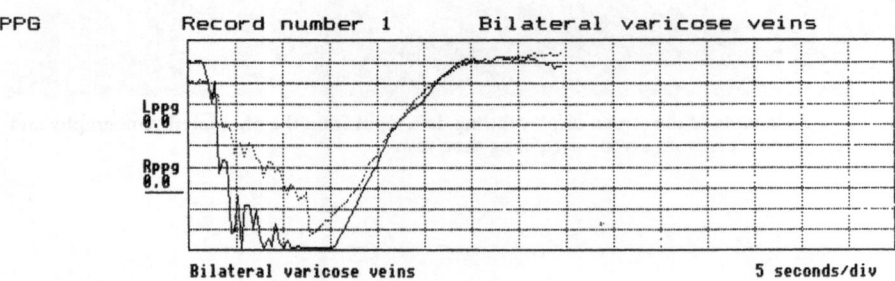

    Bilateral varicose veins   5 seconds/div

Photoplethysmography RIGHT LEFT
Refilling time (secs)   16.3   13.1

PPG   Record number 2   Bilateral deep venous insuff.

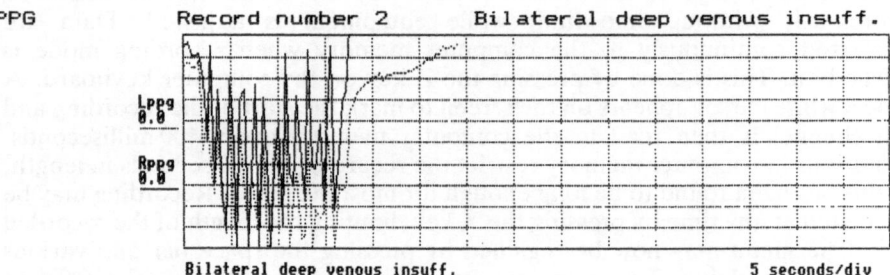

    Bilateral deep venous insuff.   5 seconds/div

Photoplethysmography RIGHT LEFT
Refilling time (secs)   0.8   4.5

Fig. 6.11. A demonstration report from the photoplethysmography program for venous refilling tests.

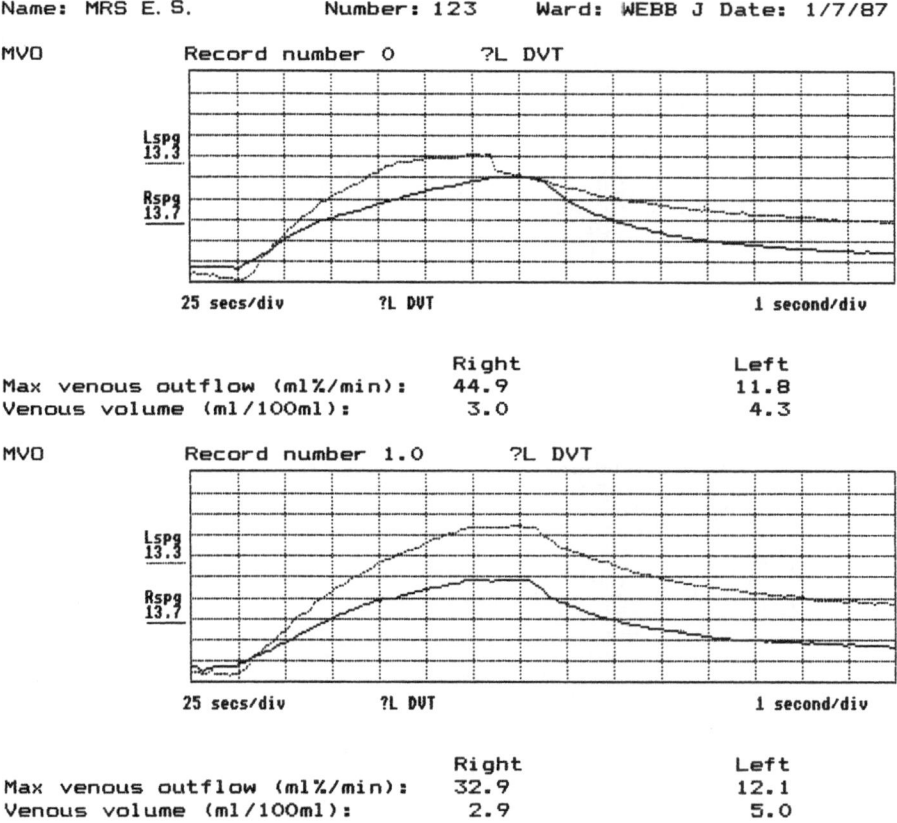

Fig. 6.12. A report from the venous outflow program.

Analysis of Data

A variety of different configurations of traces are obtained as can be seen from Figs 6.11–6.13. Various steps are required in the analysis of this data. Firstly the various parts of the traces must be recognised, unsatisfactory data rejected and further analysis prevented. If insufficient change in level is obtained for any trace the information that it contains will be unreliable and this initial check is made in all analyses. Most traces rely on a starting level being established and the programs check that this is stable so that a baseline may be gauged.

In the case of PPG and foot volumetry programs the section of the trace to be analysed is the rising phase following exercise. In both cases this should be a constantly rising phase and the programs search for a period of 2 seconds in which the level rises continuously. This is then taken as the start of the section on which calculations will be performed, and the initial 1 second of the data is

THE MIDDLESEX HOSPITAL
Vascular Laboratory
Venous Assessment

Name: FRED BLOGGS   Number: 123456   Ward: LATYMER   Date: 1/11/87

FVOL   Record number 0   NORMAL LEGS

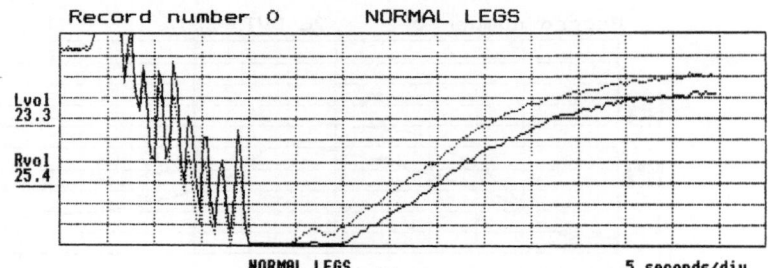

                    NORMAL LEGS   5 seconds/div

Foot volumetry   RIGHT LEFT
Refilling time (secs) 66.1   73.2
Return time (secs)   44.8   50.8
Volume change (ml)   19.8   21.7

FVOL   Record number 1   R&L VARICOSE VEINS

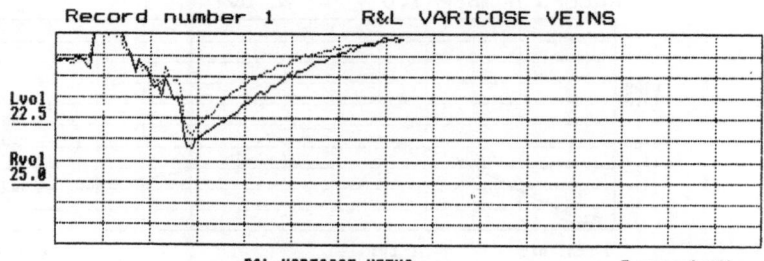

                R&L VARICOSE VEINS   5 seconds/div

Foot volumetry   RIGHT LEFT
Refilling time (secs) 20.7   12.7
Return time (secs)   14.4   10.4
Volume change (ml)   7.9   6.8

FVOL   Record number 2   R&L DEEP VEIN REFLUX

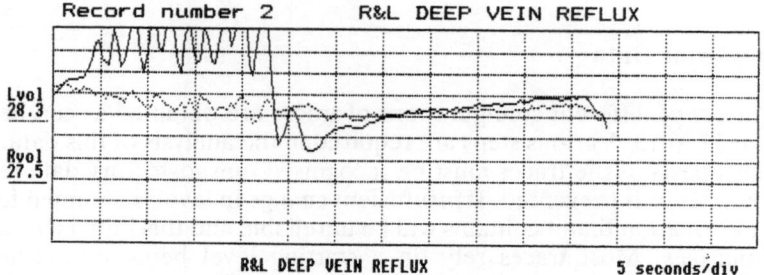

                R&L DEEP VEIN REFLUX   5 seconds/div

Foot volumetry   RIGHT LEFT
Refilling time (secs)   0.0   0.0
Return time (secs)   0.0   0.0
Volume change (ml)   0.0   0.0

Fig. 6.13. A report from the foot volumetry program.

discarded as being unreliable, since it falls in the transition phase between exercise and rest. The foot volumetry traces usually follow a reasonably mono-exponential recovery phase and an equation of the form:

$$Y = A(1 - e^{-Bt})$$

(where Y is the transducer output voltage, t is time, and A and B are the coefficients) is fitted to the data using a least squares method. This removes the irregularities in the curve and allows calculation of the recovery time (to 95 % of the initial resting value) as well as the volume change of the foot. The PPG curves vary considerably, but were initially fitted to a mono-exponential curve. It became apparent that this was frequently not very satisfactory and the current programs use an equation of the form:

$$Y = A + B/t + C/t^2 + D/t^3 + E/t^4$$

that is, a fourth order inverse polynomial equation. The fit is achieved by compiling simultaneous equations and solving these by Gaussian elimination. The equations obtained remove the irregularities of the curve and achieve an adequate fit in most instances. The equations are solved by induction to determine the time when the computed curve crosses the level corresponding to 95 % of the starting level.

Despite the apparent complexity of these techniques they are entirely objective and can be carried out in a period of 5–30 seconds for each curve, depending on the amount of recorded data.

The venous outflow traces contain an essentially mono-exponential emptying curve to which an equation of the form:

$$Y = 1/Ae^{-t}$$

is fitted by least squares, with excellent correlation in most cases. Again the parameters of venous volume may be calculated with ease from the equation.

Report Generation

The venous plethysmography traces are reproduced on the final report using a dot matrix printer. This was decided upon in preference to the plotter because the length of most of the plethysmography files would have meant frequent re-loading of paper, since this device can hold only one sheet of paper at one time. The present generation of programs will report all the files that may be accommodated on one side of a disc (eleven files) each of which may hold sixteen sets of traces, a total of 176 traces altogether, without the intervention of the operator. Each trace is first drawn on the computer screen, and then copied to the printer using a machine code screen dump. The data are then analysed and the derived results copied to the printer using conventional printing mode. This is repeated for each set of traces in the file, fitting three sets of traces on each A4 page plus the title and footer lines.

Software Techniques

The display of plethysmograph data necessitated a horizontally scrolling screen. The same considerations come into effect as in the Doppler software described above. The problem of moving large areas of memory about in order to achieve scrolling was again a problem. The possibility of scrolling the whole screen, which can be achieved by direct commands to the VDU controller chip, was discarded since useful information of the graph axes would be rapidly scrolled out of sight. The solution we have used is to scroll the area of the screen required by 8 pixels horizontally once per second when required. This does produce a slightly jerky motion, but is acceptable. The axes are left in their original positions so that calibration data and instructions are not lost. The scroll requires that about 16 K of memory are moved and takes a quarter of a second. The basis of this is uncomplicated. The layout of memory used for the display is very similar to that described for mode 0 screens in the Doppler software section. In screen mode 1 used by this part of the program, each byte represents 4 pixels. Each pair of bits selects one of four colours for each pixel. They are laid out in a similar fashion to mode 0, that is with successive groups of eight bytes in the same vertical column, then moving horizontally to the next column. A scroll to the left is achieved by moving the screen contents down memory. Moving it 8 locations will cause a movement of 4 pixels, moving 16 locations will scroll 8 pixels. The latter was selected to avoid too frequent scrolling of the screen. The 8 pixels at the left of the area within the axes of the graph are not scrolled, since that would over-write the axes. They are instead simply changed to reflect the contents of the columns to their right as part of the scroll. The right edge of the screen is cleared and new sections of the grid drawn using standard BBC BASIC plot commands. During scrolling, the traces are always plotted on the same piece of the screen, and then scrolled to the left. This places no limit on the period for which a trace may be viewed. The routine to achieve this was written in machine code, and occupies the 256 bytes of RAM just below the screen area (&2FOO–&2FFF). The BBC Master computer now incorporates such routines as part of the VDU driver software, and these may be called from a VDU command.

Data are saved in this system in a rather similar way to that in the Doppler software. A memory buffer is reserved between locations &2BOO and &2EFF. Locations &2EFD–&2EFF are used to store any calibration factors required for the quantitative tests. The remainder of the buffer area holds data read from the A/D convertors. In the original system, designed to read and display four channels of data simultaneously, the data are held as groups of four bytes. Each group holds the data from each channel read at one time, with room for 254 sets of data. The data are read in at 400 millisecond intervals, this having been found to give sufficient resolution. In a similar way to the Doppler software, the memory buffer is continuously updated with the incoming data irrespective of whether it is required. The traces are also displayed at the same time. The start of recording is selected when the user presses the Z key on the computer keyboard. The current writing position in the memory buffer is transferred to two bytes just below the buffer. At the end of the recording session (up to 100 seconds later), when the user presses the X key, the finish location of valid data is stored in the adjacent two bytes. Software checks are made to ensure that the start of the recording is not over-written should record mode be left on for more than 100 seconds. The complete set of data is the entire contents of the buffer and the pointers to the start and finish of valid data. These are saved together on disc for future analysis or display. The input section of software will only display 35 seconds and the analysis section 70 seconds of the data in the buffer at one time, although the analysis software may examine all of the recorded data. Therefore it is essential for the programs to be able to identify the start and end of valid data. This technique of using a buffer with pointers makes it simple to delete a trace: all that is necessary is to re-start the recording by pressing Z again to update the start location and X when the recording is finished. This facilitates the acquisition of traces where many data may have to be discarded.

Some difficulty was encountered during program development because of the memory limitations of BBC Model B microcomputers, which have as little as 5 K bytes of memory available in the higher resolution screen modes (modes 0–2). The programs were divided up into sections and made to call each other. The analysis program, 8 K bytes long, would not fit in memory in mode 0 which was required for high resolution screen dumping. Since only half the screen was used to draw the display, the other half was blanked and used to hold the program! These techniques are now no longer necessary with the availability of BBC microcomputers which have a full 30 K bytes of memory in all screen modes.

Database Information Storage

A small database program for the BBC microcomputer has been used to hold the details of all patients examined in the laboratory and also generates a front sheet for the reports in which data are summarised along with any comments and conclusions.

Portable Vascular Laboratory

In order that we should have a set of equipment to take to patients in the clinic or ward, a microcomputer has been mounted on a trolley along with a PPG machine and a Doppler ultrasound device. The computer has been equipped with the appropriate interface and programs have been transferred to ROMs (Read Only Memories), chips which plug into the computer and hold information even when the power is turned off. The programs are then already present in the machine when it is turned on and need only be started by the correct commands for the unit to be operational (Fig. 6.14).

Moving software to ROMs is a technique that may be useful for frequently used programs that are infrequently updated. The BBC microcomputer allows ROMs to be used as a filing system so that data or programs may be accessed as if they were on a floppy disc or network fileserver. In this particular computer the programs need not necessarily run as machine code from the ROM, which would have been difficult on this occasion in view of the mathematical gymnastics necessary to perform fourth order polynomial regression! Use of ROMs in this way is not completely straightforward since the BBC microcomputer has the facilities to accommodate up to 16 such ROMs in the same 16 K of memory space! Each must contain a small section of machine code which must arbitrate with the opening system to declare its capabilities and contents. Details

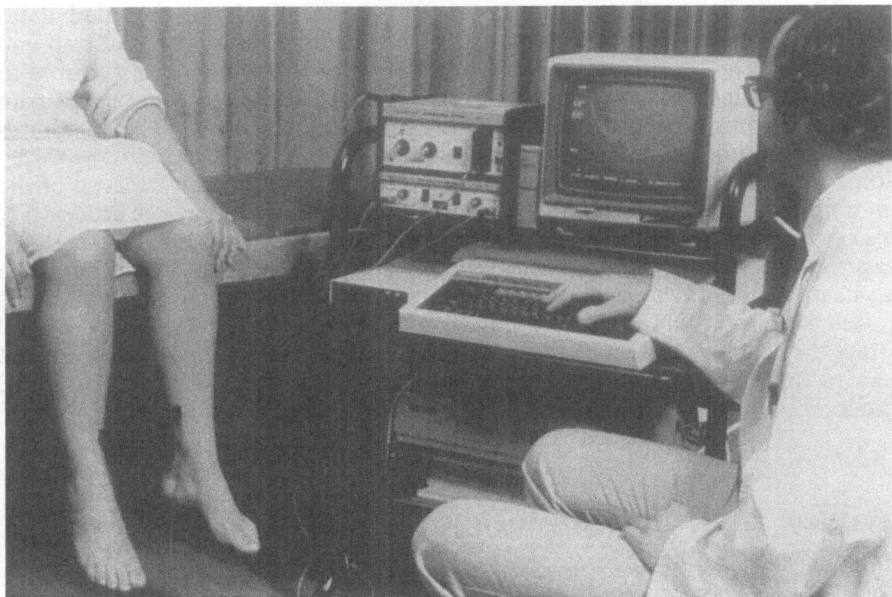

Fig. 6.14. The portable version of the computerised vascular laboratory in use for the diagnosis of venous disorders of the lower limb.

of this may be obtained in reference from the standard reference books [1,2]. The ROM filing system uses the same data format as the cassette filing system, with data broken up into blocks, usually of 256 bytes. Each block has a header which as well as containing the filename also contains error check characters, the cyclical redundancy check (CRC) bytes. These ensure that data integrity is not lost between storage and retrieval. A program was written to create complete files ready for burning into EPROMs (erasable and electronically programmable ROMs). This requests the names of files to be included in the ROM, and checks their presence on the disc in the current drive. It then breaks each into 256 byte blocks, generates a header for each including the CRC bytes, and writes the results to another disc file. Finally a ROM header is added to the start of the file so that the completed ROM will announce itself correctly to the computer operating system. A commercially available EPROM progammer is used to copy the file into EPROM before it is installed in the computer.

This technique has been used in the portable system to avoid the necessity of having a system disc and an extra disc drive. The programs are already present at power-on and may be started by auto-booting the ROM filing system which is achieved by the unlikely combination of pressing the shift, delete and break keys simultaneously. Programs load reasonably rapidly but somewhat more slowly than they would from disc. This is especially noticeable on the Master series machines. Once in operation the software functions in precisely the same way as on disc, but without the need for frequent disc access. Only the trace data are held on disc in order to make a permanent record of a particular examination.

Conclusions

Over 1000 patients have been examined using this laboratory arrangement in the past two years and it now takes only 30–40 minutes for most examinations. Preparation of reports is usually a simple task since correctly annotated traces are already available for examination. The microcomputer considerably facilitates the assessment of patients with both arterial and venous problems.

References

1 The advanced user guide to the BBC microcomputer (1981). Acorn, Cambridge
2 BBC microcomputer reference manual (1984). Acorn, Cambridge

7 Microcomputer-Assisted Analysis of Audiological Test Data

S.L. Smith, M.C. Fairhurst, S.W. Kelly and J.S.R. Baxter

Introduction

Hearing tests are routinely performed in hospitals, out-patient clinics, schools (in mass screening programmes) and other locations. Though testing procedures can vary and can be of varying degrees of sophistication, the most commonly adopted is the standard pure-tone test, in which the patient is exposed to a range of single tones at various frequencies and intensities and is required to acknowledge their perception, allowing the clinician to obtain a broad picture of hearing performance over the frequency spectrum of clinical interest.

This type of test is invaluable for screening and for preliminary clinical diagnostic procedures. Despite the relative simplicity of the test itself, the interpretation of the results requires experience and clinical expertise. Even when these are readily available, the changing characteristics of hearing with factors such as age and sex and the lack of precise uniformity between individuals can often present difficulties, introducing a degree of uncertainty which contrasts with the positive benefits afforded by the simplicity of the test.

The primary objective of the work reported here is to investigate the extent to which microcomputer technology can be exploited to create a better match between convenience and simplicity in the testing of hearing on the one hand, and speed and reliability in the interpretation of results obtained on the other. The approach taken was to work towards the design and implementation of a prototype microcomputer-based system which will receive data from a hearing test and generate a display which both conforms to an accepted standard representation of hearing performance and which gives immediate help in data interpretation. Related questions tackled include aspects of man–machine interaction within the system (particularly from the point of view of matching data entry to an existing environment) and the manipulation of subsidiary facilities which enhance the benefits of the system for the clinician.

The next section introduces the background to audiological measurement (with particular reference to pure-tone hearing testing) and describes current clinical practice. A critical analysis of current audiological methods is then given and this leads to a proposal for the design of a microcomputer-based system which offers the possibility of improving these procedures. The development of the proposed system is then described and this is followed by an assessment of the system and its performance in a clinical environment.

Thus the work reported here tackles the basic issues in clinical and technological practice which underlie the design, implementation and assessment of a system to meet the criteria described above. As will be seen, these considerations lead to the development of a working prototype which is currently in regular use at the Kent and Canterbury Hospital and which has been received with enthusiasm by the staff there.

Audiological Testing and Test Procedures

It is self-evident that the reason for testing a person's hearing is to detect any defect that may be present and to diagnose its cause so that treatment may be prescribed where necessary. A principal tool in hearing tests is the clinical audiogram, and its generation is a well-established procedure which is outlined below.

Before a hearing test proceeds, the patient's ears are checked for any large amounts of ear wax which could cause misleading results [1]. The patient then sits in a sound-proofed booth and is fitted with a pair of headphones, which is connected to an audiometer, situated outside of the box. The audiometer is a device which is capable of creating pure-tones over a range of frequencies and intensities (a pure-tone being a sound consisting of one frequency only with no overtones). These pure-tones are presented one at a time to either the left or right ear of the patient via the headphones and at the discretion of the clinician. The patient is able to acknowledge the hearing of a tone, usually by pressing a push-button switch which lights a lamp on the audiometer. This is not the only method of acknowledging perception of tones in clinical audiology, the raising of a hand or finger is another common approach, and in some cases can provide more information to the clinician about the validity of the response [2].

The intensity of the pure-tone presented to the patient is measured in decibels and in terms of a nationally accepted standard [3] which is different for each frequency tested. The national standard can be described as being the lowest intensity that can be heard by an average 18 year old person with clinically "normal" ears for a particular frequency and defines the reference level of 0 decibels. Higher intensities of pure-tones are described by a positive measurement of greater than zero decibels, and similarly lower intensities are described by a negative measurement. It is the clinician's task to test the patient's hearing by measuring the lowest intensity level audible at each frequency that is to be tested. The patient is instructed to press the push-button switch every time a tone on the headphones is heard. The clinician then selects a frequency at which to test the ear and presents a tone at that frequency at an intensity that is easily heard by the majority of patients, usually 50 decibels. The intensity of the tone is then gradually reduced by steps of 10 decibels until the patient can no longer hear it (i.e. when the patient no longer responds) and then increased by steps of 5 decibels until its presence is registered again in the manner described above. The level is then reduced in 10 dB steps and increased in 5 dB steps again, so that two agreeing ascending readings can be obtained.

Both ears are tested separately over a certain set of frequencies, which in the majority of clinical situations consist of the test frequencies 0.125 kHz, 0.25 kHz, 0.5 kHz, 1.0 kHz, 2.0 kHz, 4.0 kHz and 8.0 kHz, while occasionally frequencies of 1.5 kHz, 3.0 kHz and 6.0 kHz are also tested. The lowest intensity of a pure-tone that can be heard by a patient at a particular frequency is known as the hearing threshold level for that frequency.

It is worth noting that, despite the apparent simplicity of the testing procedure, its effective execution can only be guaranteed when under the supervision of a skilled and qualified clinician (see, for example, [2]). Furthermore, it should be pointed out that pure-tone audiological testing, though perhaps the most frequently carried out, is nevertheless not the only hearing test used for diagnostic purposes [4].

Recording of Hearing Threshold Levels

In the testing of a person's hearing, as described above, as each hearing threshold level is measured it is recorded on a special graph called an audiogram, one example of which is shown in Fig. 7.1. As can be seen, the audiogram contains two subgraphs, one for each ear. The frequencies at which the ear is tested are marked out along the X-axis of the graph, and the intensity at which these tones are produced are marked out along the Y-axis. It is therefore possible for the clinician to mark on the graph the lowest intensity tone audible by the patient for each frequency of interest as the test proceeds. In the example shown in Fig. 7.1, the points on the graph corresponding to the left ear have been marked with an X character, and those for the right ear with an O character. It is common clinical practice to record the response of the left ear on the right hand of the audiogram and the response of the right ear on the left, so that when a specialist is facing the patient, the appropriate graph on the audiogram corresponds to the correct side of the patient as seen by the clinician.

Once the audiogram has been completed by the clinician, the patient is usually sent immediately to the specialist. Equipped with the audiogram, the patient's records and his own experience, the specialist has the task of analysing the results.

Analysis of the Audiogram

The first thing the specialist has to take account of when analysing an audiogram is the patient's age, as a person's hearing naturally deteriorates as he gets older.

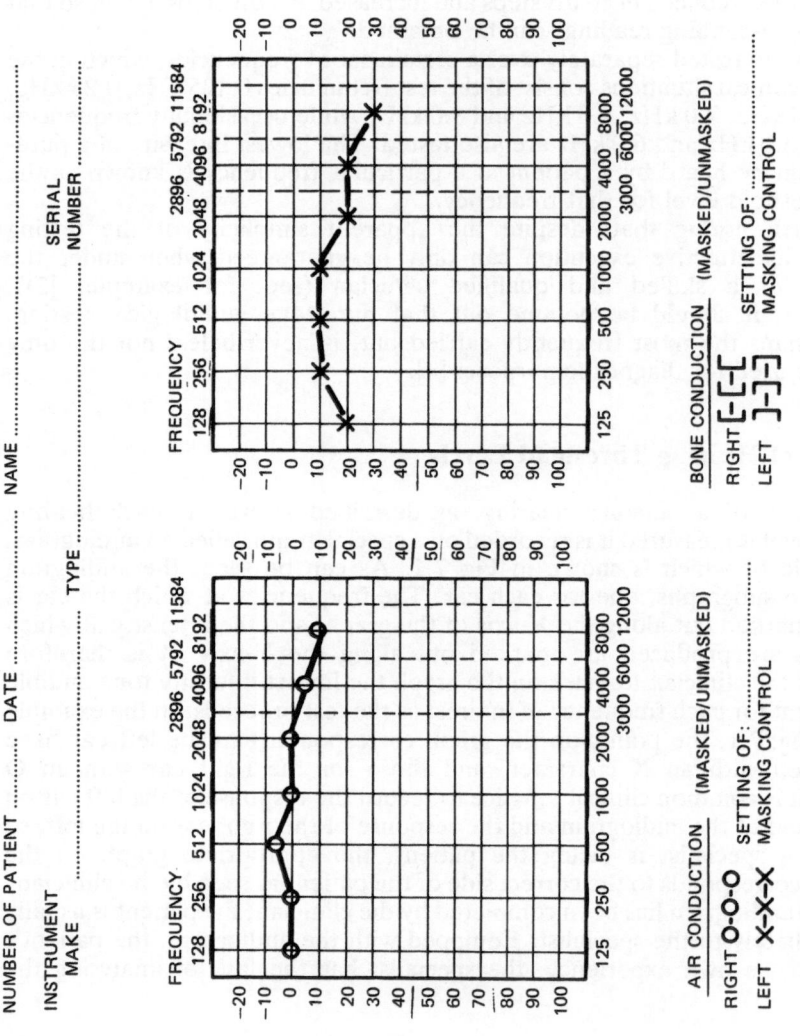

Fig. 7.1. Standard clinical audiogram.

This is a condition which is independent of any clinical disorder and is known as presbyacusis [5].

Presbyacusis

The existence of presbyacusis has been recognised for many years and several surveys have been made in this country to assess its effect on hearing in relation to age. Generally, for a person with clinically normal ears, the effect of presbyacusis should only start to become evident at about 40 to 50 years of age when a noticeable decline in perception of sound, especially in the higher frequencies, will be apparent. What is important is for the specialist to be able to decide whether any hearing loss experienced is due solely to presbyacusis or whether some other disorder is present. Currently, the specialist usually only has a set of tables, derived on a statistical basis, stating the "expected" pure-tone threshold levels for a patient of a specified age and sex over a range of sampled frequencies. From these tables it is possible to check each of the responses on the audiogram to see how it compares with the expected figures.

Once presbyacusis has been accounted for, it is possible to analyse the audiogram for other indications of defects such as noise-induced deafness, the loss of hearing due to prolonged exposure to high intensities of noise such as that found in heavy industry and so on.

Observed Problems in Current Practice

Several problems are frequently encountered in the present system of testing and assessing a person's hearing when the standard approach described above is adopted. They may be summarised as:

1. A patient's hearing threshold levels are plotted by hand in ink on paper audiograms. Once completed, the audiogram often contains mistakes and subsequently corrected early estimations of threshold levels which can lead to misinterpretation of the results. An actual clinical example of such a confused audiogram is shown in Fig. 7.2.

2. As stated above, once the audiogram has been completed by the clinician, the patient is sent directly to the specialist. This illustrates a lack of interaction between the clinician and the specialist which could lead to the loss of information that cannot be expressed on audiogram cards presently used in clinical practice.

3. When the specialist receives the audiogram, no analysis of the results has been made, and specifically the evaluation of the effect of presbyacusis, which need not be a specialised task, has not been performed. It remains the task of the specialist with the aid of only numerical tables and experience, to allow for the effects of presbyacusis and thus detect any other defects that may be present. There is considerable scope for error in this operation as the analysis described above involves the manipulation of a considerable amount of data.

4. The handling of the numerical tables outlined in the procedure above is both an inefficient and a relatively time-consuming affair.

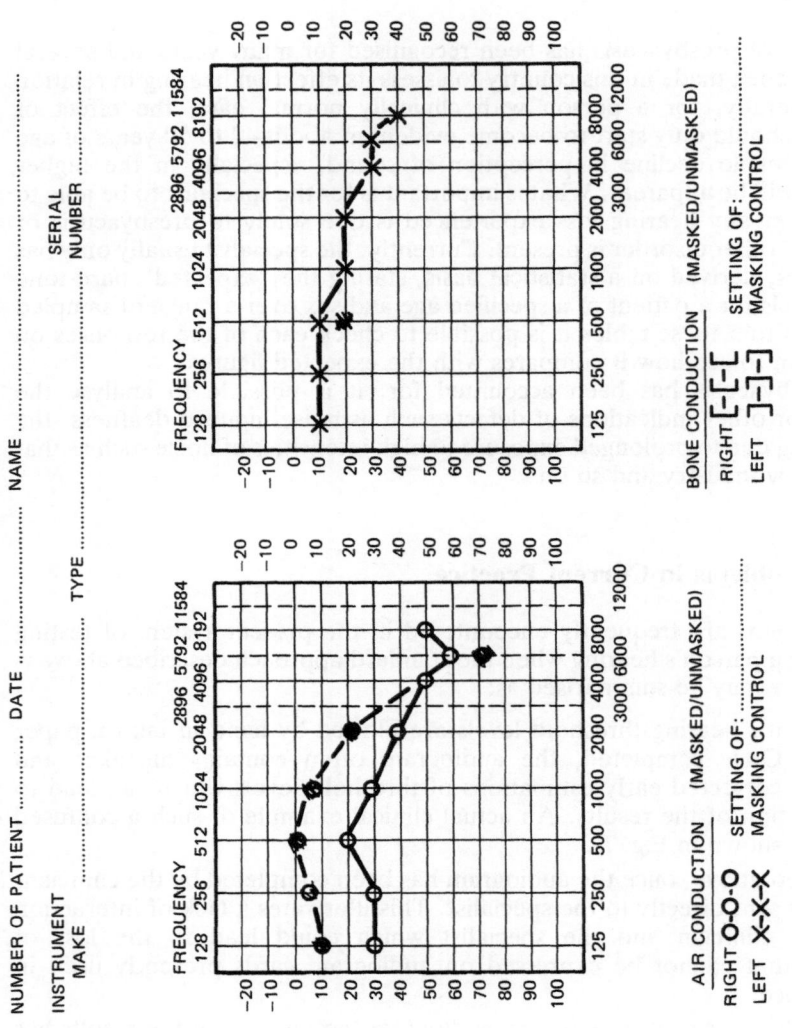

Fig. 7.2. Typically confused clinical audiogram.

System Specification, Design Objectives and Data Characteristics

As a consequence of the arguments described and the assessment of current clinical practice noted above, and in consultation with the staff of the Kent and Canterbury Hospital Audiology Department, it became clear that there was significant scope for the investigation of the design and implementation of a microcomputer-based system to aid clinical audiological testing. More specifically, a number of important design criteria were identified, and have become the principal objectives of the research project described here.

The design of a microcomputer-based system to address the problem areas noted above offers several significant advantages, including the following:

1. A microcomputer can have a good graphics capability which would be very suitable for the presentation of visual/graphical data such as the audiogram.

2. Computers are by their very nature extremely efficient at handling numerical data and performing operations on them.

3. In using a microcomputer the input of data can be more precise and checking can be made for obvious errors.

4. Microcomputers are relatively cheap and reliable pieces of equipment.

5. Data can be easily stored and accessed. This is true of the mathematical data required for the analysis of audiograms and also of data relating to individual patients.

Consequently, it is possible to formulate a specification for the implementation of a microcomputer-based system to aid clinical audiological testing, which should meet the following criteria:

1. It should allow the input and recording of audiological data resulting from hearing tests in a manner which will reduce the possibility of errors present in manual transcription.

2. It should facilitate the presentation of the data in a manner that will be clear and not open to misinterpretation, yet provide at least as much information as the current audiogram does.

3. It should have a speed of response which does not conflict with current data entry procedures and operational practices.

4. It should perform any routine, non-specialist analysis on the data which does not involve interpretation requiring the experience of a specialist. The assessment of the effect of presbyacusis is particularly relevant here.

5. It should provide a means of interaction which is acceptable to non-specialist staff in a busy clinical environment.

Although significant technical problems at the level of data manipulation and software engineering have to be tackled, from a long-term and practical point of view, the last of the criteria specified above is by far the most important. It is vital that new equipment should be acceptable to non-specialist staff, not just in terms of its technical capabilities, but also in terms of the ease with which it can be assimilated and incorporated in a familiar and established pattern of working.

Data Characteristics

As described earlier, in analysing a person's hearing it is necessary to take account of the effect of presbyacusis in order to detect any defects that may be present. In the microcomputer-based system outlined above, it is proposed that such analysis should be performed automatically. However, in order to perform this type of processing the effect of presbyacusis must be expressible numerically.

Numerical Representation of the Effect of Presbyacusis

The effect of presbyacusis can be represented numerically by the results that would be obtained in testing the hearing of an average and clinically normal patient of a specified age and sex. In other words, presbyacusis is the naturally occurring effect of age alone on the human ear, involving no other factors. Consequently its effect can be studied by the measurement of clinically "normal" ears. To illustrate this, Fig. 7.3 shows the effect that presbyacusis would have, represented numerically, on clinically normal ears of a man at the ages 20, 40 and 60 years which have been tested at the frequency of 2 kHz. As can be seen, at the age of 20 years, presbyacusis has no effect, as the hearing threshold is 0 decibels, the accepted average norm. However, the hearing

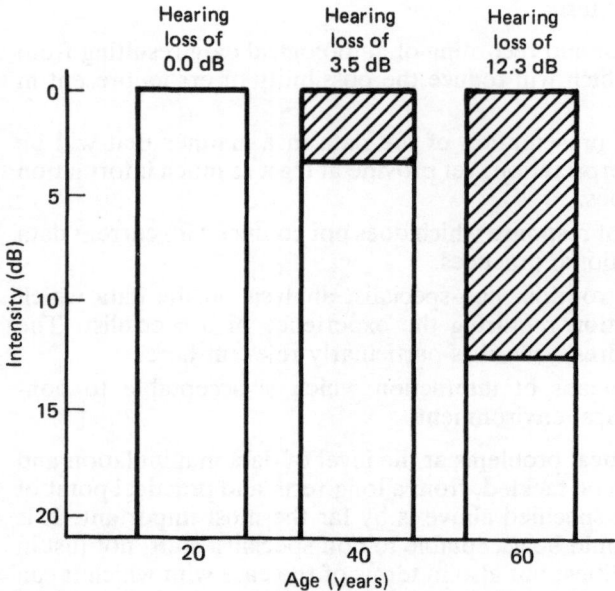

Fig. 7.3. Numerical effect of presbyacusis on hearing response with age. The clear areas on the histograms indicate hearing ability and the hatched areas indicate hearing loss.

threshold levels for ears of persons aged 40 and 60 years show the effect of presybacusis which has been represented numerically as a hearing loss of 3.5 decibels and 12.3 decibels respectively.

It can be seen from this example how valuable the numerical representation of presbyacusis can be in assessing whether or not a person's hearing is normal. The source of data used to illustrate the effect of presbyacusis numerically is from one of several surveys conducted into the hearing response of a population not experiencing any clinical disorder. The report presents hearing thresholds as a set of tables which have been constructed with data from statistical surveys on the effects of presbyacusis conducted by Robinson and Sutton [6]. The data from the survey were used to derive equations which enabled the calculation of a comprehensive set of hearing threshold levels. These threshold levels are those that can be expected from a clinically normal ear for specified test frequencies and in relation to a patient's age and sex.

The frequencies at which threshold levels are provided are 0.125 kHz, 0.25 kHz, 0.5 kHz, 1.0 kHz, 1.5 kHz, 2.0 kHz, 3.0 kHz, 4.0 kHz, 6.0 kHz, and 8.0 kHz. Different tables are provided for males and females, and each cover the ages of 20 to 70 years. Statistical deviations from the norm are also provided and cover ±1 and ±2 standard deviations. These tables are sufficient to assess the hearing threshold levels provided by a person of a particular age and sex, but the volume of the data prevents the direct storage of this information on a typical microcomputer such as that used in this project, the BBC Microcomputer.

Ten tables in all were needed for this assessment. Each table consists of hearing threshold levels at 10 different tested frequencies for all ages between 20 and 70 years, giving 510 threshold levels per table. This gives a grand total of 5100 threshold levels for the ten tables and would account for over 100 K of memory, if stored directly. The BBC model B and B+ Micros do not have this amount of RAM so data would have to be continuously read from disc or other backing store. This is not a satisfactory solution as it not only makes a backing store for the system mandatory, but it is also a very time-consuming method of data retrieval. It was therefore necessary to compress the tables by using the set of equations and dependent tables of constants which were originally used to construct the tables. The data generated by the implementation of the above equations on the BBC Micro was compared with the existing tables and it was discovered that the difference between the two was negligible and certainly within the tolerances required by this project.

System Description

A fundamental objective of the project reported here is to examine ways in which microcomputer-based systems might be used to present and analyse audiological data extracted from a conventional pure-tone audiogram measurement. In this section, the specification and implementation of such a system is described. A consideration of methods for data input to the system is then described and some preliminary clinical trials at the Audiology Department of Kent and Canterbury Hospital are assessed in the following section.

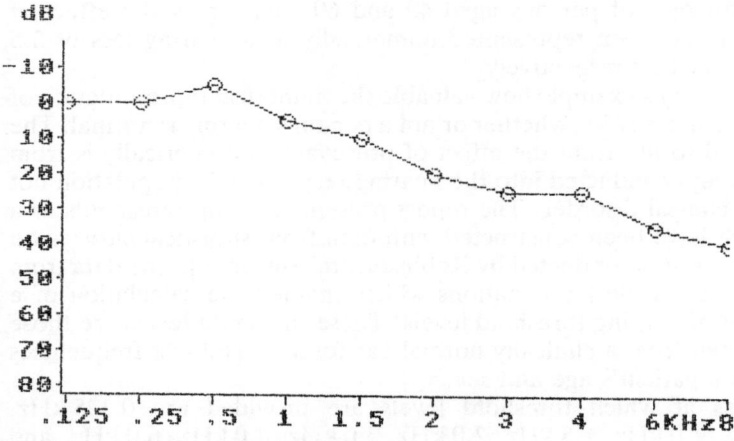

Fig. 7.4.   Screen dump of basic audiogram.

Data Displays

System development proceeded through a number of stages as designs were refined and as the dynamic process of assessment and clinical trial progressed. The purpose of the system is to present a graphical representation of a clinical audiogram on the screen of a BBC Microcomputer or, more precisely, to use computer graphics to draw an audiogram similar to those used in audiology clinics, of which an example was shown in Fig. 7.1. The BBC Microcomputer was chosen as the host for the system principally because of the good graphics that are provided. Fig. 7.4 shows the audiogram produced using mode 1 of BBC Micro graphics, making some four colours available with high resolution. High resolution in this context is defined as 320×256 picture elements (pixels). As can be seen in Fig. 7.4, an attempt has been made to represent the audiogram as a conventional graph to aid clarity. Both the frequency and intensity at which pure-tones are generated are presented in the same manner as would be found on a conventional audiogram. The hearing threshold levels have been presented in a simple manner on the graph as dots connected with straight lines and, again, this is how hearing threshold levels are presented clinically. The speed at which the BBC Micro generated the audiogram was impressive, being less than a second in all.

Data Analysis

This section describes how analysis is performed on the audiogram with particular reference to the effect of presbyacusis. We have already shown how the effect of presbyacusis could be represented numerically, and have described how tables containing this numerical representation had been compressed so that they could be loaded into and subsequently accessed from a microcomputer. The first design principle was to consider the optimum way in which the effect of presbyacusis could be represented graphically on the audiogram. The second

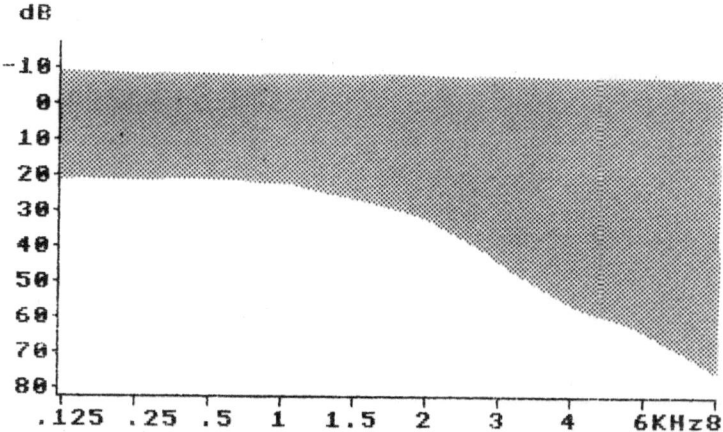

Fig. 7.5. Screen dump of audiogram illustrating normal band.

problem for consideration was how the numerical data could be manipulated to produce this graphical representation.

As described earlier, for a person of given age and sex, a set of hearing threshold levels which would represent the effect of presbyacusis can be generated numerically. Statistical deviations of these mean figures, specifically the ±1 and ±2 standard deviations can also be generated. After consultation with the specialist at the Audiology Department at Kent and Canterbury Hospital, it was agreed that any hearing threshold levels resulting from a hearing test that lie between ±2 standard deviations of the mean figures would be considered as normal. Normal is used in this sense to mean a deviation from the accepted norm that should not generally (other things being equal) give any cause for concern. It was therefore decided that this range of normality should be represented on the audiogram in a manner which would indicate clearly whether the recorded thresholds from a hearing test were in fact normal or not.

In order to achieve this, it was decided to represent this range of normality as a (red) band on the audiogram as illustrated in Fig. 7.5. The hearing threshold levels can then be plotted as a line which is superimposed on this normal band. This enables the classification of hearing threshold levels instantly as normal or abnormal depending on whether or not they lie within the (red) band. This is illustrated in Figs 7.6 and 7.7. The colour red was chosen to represent the normal band to exploit the natural responsiveness of the human eye and it contrasts well between the white hearing-threshold line and the black background.

An interesting point to note here is the manner in which the effect of presbyacusis on a person's hearing was represented graphically in the program described above. The desired effect, as stated earlier, was to cancel out the effect of presbyacusis so an analysis of the audiogram could be conducted without having to take account of this feature. It was suggested that the straight forward subtraction of the expected hearing threshold levels (i.e. those illustrating the expected effect of presbyacusis provided by a survey) from those of the patient's hearing level thresholds would provide the desired filtering. This, however, was considered to distort the audiogram making further analysis

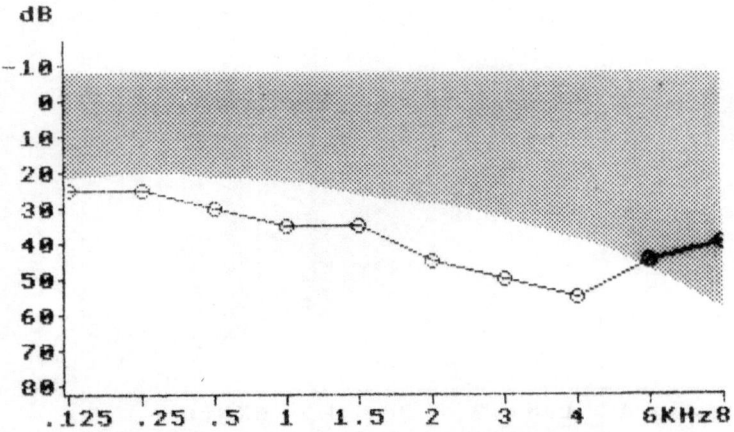

Fig. 7.6. Audiogram illustrating a normal hearing response.

difficult, so the method of superimposing the patient's threshold levels with the expected levels was implemented. This has the distinct advantage that when a patient's hearing threshold levels are presented the specialist knows that they are always the original responses and have not been manipulated in any way. It is also easier to assess the difference between the two sets of thresholds when they are superimposed than when one has been subtracted from the other.

It can be concluded that the effect of presbyacusis in the form of a normal band can be represented graphically on a microcomputer in a manner that gives clear comparison with hearing threshold levels from a patient's hearing test.

In order to produce an audiogram with a normal band representing the effect of presbyacusis for a particular patient, it is necessary for the system to be given information about the patient's age and sex. Similarly, if the computer is then to superimpose on a normal range band the patient's specific audiogram, the hearing threshold level measurements must be input to the computer. The

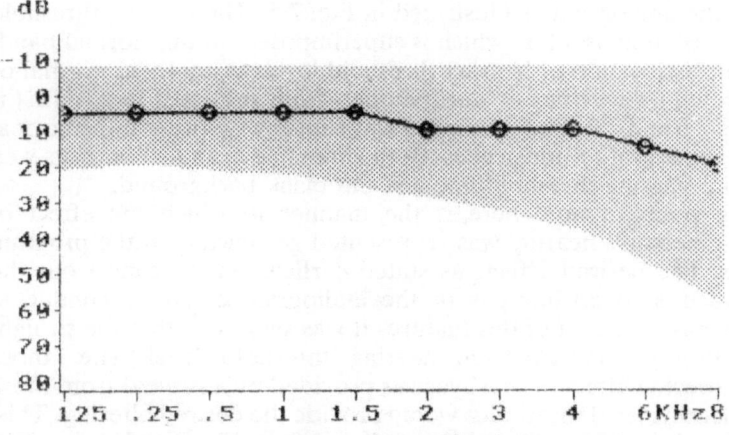

Fig. 7.7. Audiogram illustrating an abnormal hearing response.

program was developed to facilitate entry of this information before any attempt to produce an audiogram was made. This development is discussed later along with other data-input considerations of the system, but in the initial version data was input in response to a series of questionnaire type questions.

Once these data have been acquired by the microcomputer, it is possible for the screen to be cleared. The audiogram for the right ear of the patient is first displayed, superimposed with a normal band representing the effect of presbyacusis as described and illustrated in the previous section. In addition a title in the top right-hand corner of the screen is provided to indicate to which ear the audiogram relates.

The bottom third of the screen has been utilised to present data on the patient. This is illustrated in Fig. 7.8. The data consist of the patient's name, age, sex and the list of hearing threshold levels provided for the ear which is currently the subject of the display. It was thought that this information would prove valuable for cross reference, especially if a hard copy of the screen display is subsequently produced.

In order to provide a figure of merit indicating a patient's hearing performance after having been tested, a figure labelled as deviation, measured in decibels, is also provided. This figure is an assessment of how far the patient's hearing threshold levels for that ear deviate from the expected levels provided by the survey tables employed – i.e. the centre of the normal band. This figure was calculated by subtracting the expected hearing level threshold from the patient's hearing level threshold for each sampling frequency in the speech range. For clinical purposes, the speech range covers the 1 kHz to 4 kHz frequency band [7]. Each of the resulting values that are greater than the +2 standard deviations of the norm are summed and the total figure presented as the deviation. This

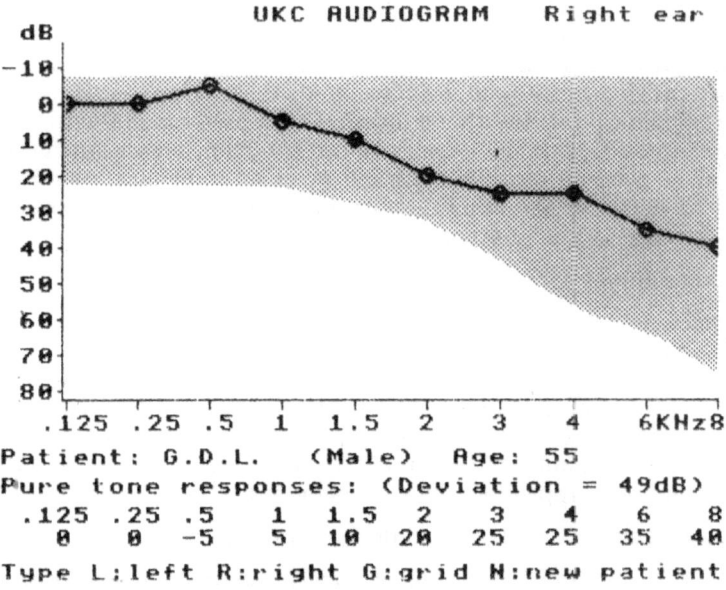

Fig. 7.8. Audiogram with displayed patient data.

figure therefore gives an indication in decibels of how the patient's hearing for that ear relates to the expected response for a patient of their age and sex. In place of this deviation figure, it is possible (and may be desirable) to substitute a categorisation of the patient's hearing response as specified by the Health and Safety Executive's discussion document *Audiometry in Industry* [8].

Interactive Features

Several useful interactive facilities have been provided to make the use of the system easier and to provide more information about the patient's hearing response. These features are operated by selecting the appropriate key on the microcomputer keyboard.

L – Display left ear

This command clears the screen and presents a graphical representation of the audiogram of the left ear, superimposed on the normal band (representation of presbyacusis) is the same manner as the audiogram of the right ear was produced. A figure expressing the deviation of hearing threshold levels from the norm for the left ear is calculated and is displayed with the rest of the patient data.

R – Display right ear

This clears the screen and presents the audiogram and patient data for the right ear again. It is useful to be able to switch between the two audiograms so they may be compared. It is in this application that the fast graphics provided have proved particularly useful.

G – Superimpose grid on audiogram

This command superimposes a grid on the audiogram as illustrated in Fig. 7.9. This feature was provided so that the measurement of responses at frequencies other than those provided can easily be calculated. For example, it is not often the case in current clinical practice that a threshold is measured at a frequency of 1.5 kHz, but the intensity at which the hearing threshold line crosses the grid line at this frequency can easily be estimated and gives an indication of what the intensity might be if tested. Selecting the G command the first time provides a superimposed grid, pressing it a second time removes that grid.

E – Extend audiogram

This command causes the audiogram to be extended in the Y-axis from a limit of 80 decibels to that of 110 decibels. Any part of the threshold graph that was previously not visible, corresponding to intensities greater than 80 decibels, will now be plotted. The extension of the graph in this manner dictates that the patient data are cleared, as the space that they usually occupy is required. On the second use of the command, the extended section of the graph is cleared and the patient information is reprinted. This is illustrated in Figs 7.10 and 7.11.

M – Display mean and ±1 standard deviation of mean lines

On selection of this command the mean and ±1 standard deviation of the mean representation of the effect of presbyacusis are displayed as black lines on

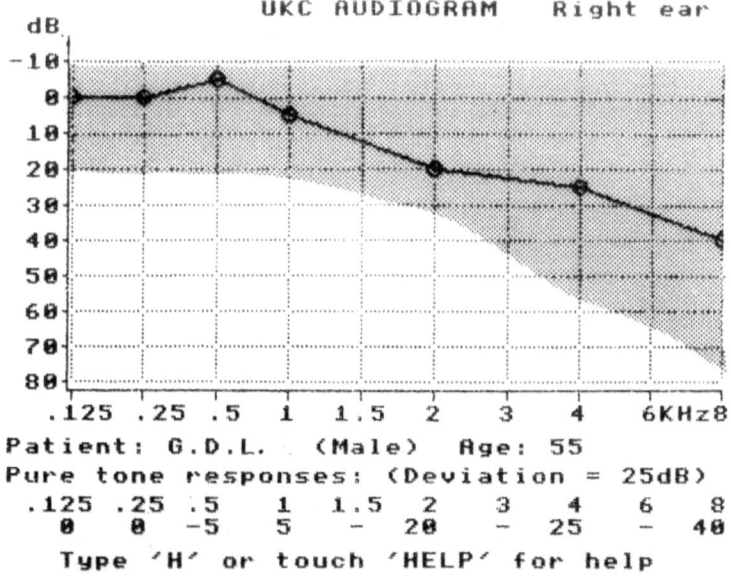

Fig. 7.9.   Audiogram illustrating superimposed grid.

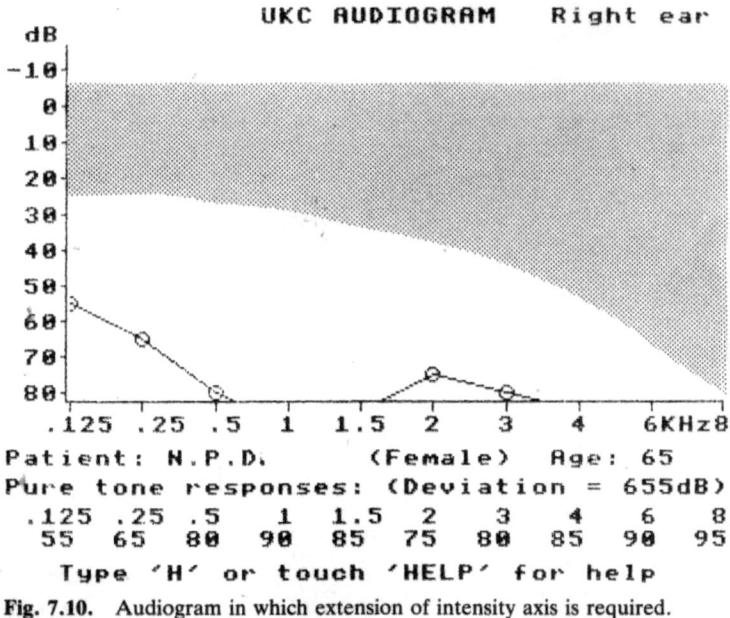

Fig. 7.10.   Audiogram in which extension of intensity axis is required.

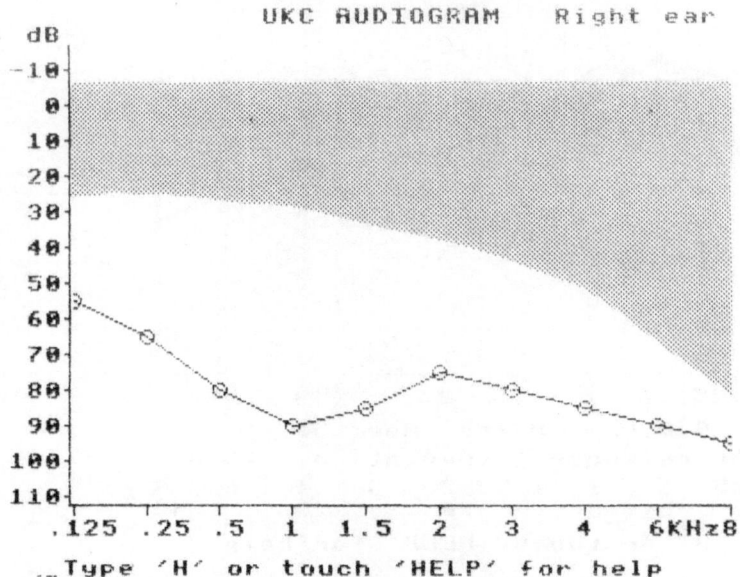

Fig. 7.11. Audiogram in extended mode.

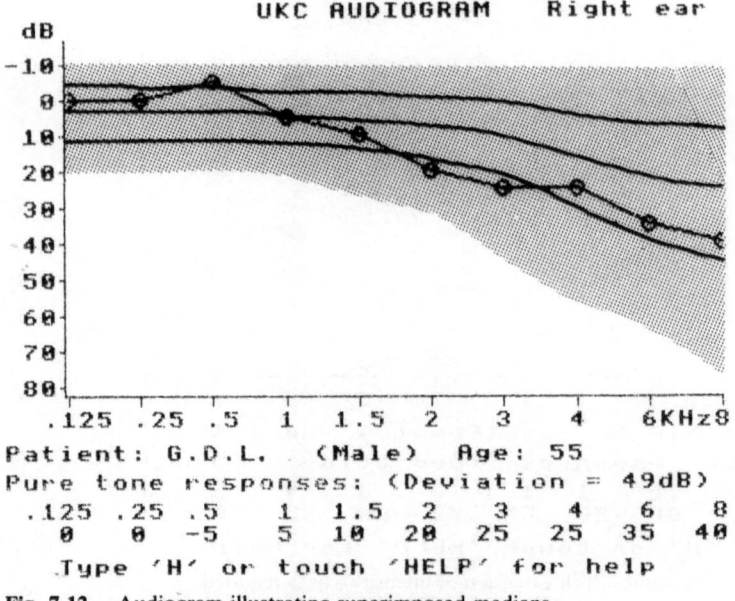

Fig. 7.12. Audiogram illustrating superimposed medians.

the red normal band as illustrated in Fig. 7.12. On successive selection of this command the mean and ±1 standard deviation lines are removed.

When the above commands were implemented it was decided that it should be possible to use either or both of the commands in conjunction with the grid facility already implemented. In any of the permutations of these three commands the hearing threshold line is always re-drawn last so it is most visible. In most cases the three commands work independently of each other.

H – Provide help information

This command clears the screen and lists each of the available command letters with a brief description of what the command does. On the subsequent selection of any key on the keyboard, the previous audiogram is re-displayed.

The provision of this type of help facility is essential if a system with so many commands is to be used in a clinical environment where the operator of the system may have only limited knowledge of computing, or where rapid acquisition of operating skills is required in order to maximise the utilisation of the system.

N – Prepare for new patient data

This command simply causes the program to clear the screen and to dispose of all information relating to the previous patient and initiates the call for prompting information for the audiogram of a new patient.

Data Input

The method employed to input data into any system is important as this can have a large influence on the ultimate success of the system. Factors such as speed, accuracy and convenience of the inputting of data are all important. The intention that the final system should be installed in a clinical environment where the staff will have a limited knowledge of computing will also have a considerable influence. For the first clinical system all data had to be entered via the keyboard of the microcomputer. When the system is initialised for a new patient the screen is cleared and the name, age and sex of the patient are then requested in the questionnaire style as follows.

Name of patient
Enter name of patient: G.D.L.

Since any text entered by the user up to a carriage return is assigned to a string variable in the program and is used only as a label to identify the data that follow any form of reference number or other identifier can therefore be used in place of the patient's name. This gives an extra degree of generality to the operation of the system.

Age of patient
Enter age of patient (0–100): 35

The age of the patient has now been requested, with an indication of the range in which the response should lie (0–100 years). The value returned by the user is accepted as a string variable so checks can be made to ensure that the value is, in fact, solely numerical and does not contain letters. Once it has been verified that a number has been returned by the user, the string variable can be converted in to the corresponding integer. Should the response either not be numerical or numerical and out of the range indicated, the above prompt is re-issued and the previous value returned is discarded.

Sex of patient

Male or Female? (M or F): F

Next the sex of the patient is requested, and as before an indication of the response expected is given (M or F). A string is subsequently accepted by the software which is then tested to see whether the first character of the string is either M or F. This allows for the full input of the words MALE or FEMALE to be accepted. Should any string be returned that does not have M or F as its first character then the prompt is re-issued and the previous reply ignored.

Hearing threshold levels of patient

Enter values for these frequencies:

Right ear
125 Hz: 0
250 Hz: 5
500 Hz: 5
1   kHz: 10
1.5 kHz: 15
2   kHz: 15
3   kHz: 25
4   kHz: 30
6   kHz: 35
8   kHz: 40

(An identical procedure is used to request and enter corresponding data for the left ear.)

The hearing threshold levels, in decibels, are now requested by the software for both the left and right ears for the frequencies listed above. The value provided is checked in a similar manner to that adopted in inputting the age of the patient, this means that the value specified is accepted as a string variable and checked before being evaluated. Should the value returned be an alphanumeric or a figure out of range then the following message is printed.

Value must be in range −10 dB to 110 dB

The prompt is then re-issued and the previous value discarded. Should the clinician not have a hearing threshold value for the frequency prompted then the RETURN key alone may be pressed, which indicates to the software that no value is available. On completion of the submission of hearing threshold levels the audiogram for the right ear is then graphically produced on the monitor screen (as described earlier). It is then possible for the user to select any one of the available commands (which were summarised above).

When this first system was developed, the amount of data entered via the keyboard was kept to a minimum. Abbreviations for commands were used to minimise input activity and only the actual figures of the hearing threshold levels were required, as the frequencies at which they were recorded were prompted by the system. Error checking was also provided to prevent simple errors caused by mistyping such as the return of an alphanumeric string instead of a figure and the presentation of figures out of range.

Following trials at the hospital, however, reservations about this method of data-entry (although the most obvious) via the keyboard of the microcomputer were expressed. The clinicians in the audiology department were neither experienced in typing nor accustomed to interaction with microcomputers. They found the use of a keyboard for entering data led to a considerable number of errors, which once submitted could not be edited. The consequence of such errors implied that all data would have to be re-input, which was not only time consuming but equally liable to error.

Two proposals were made to try and improve the situation described above:

1. It was decided to explore the potentiality of using a different method for the input of numerical data so that a keyboard need not be used. After consideration of such peripherals as light pens, touch-sensitive screens and similar devices, it was decided to consider a solution which incorporated a graphics tablet. This choice was made as it was considered that a graphics tablet is a peripheral which is potentially closest to the (currently accepted) activity of plotting an audiogram on a card.

2. Once threshold levels have been entered into the microcomputer, it should be possible to edit them so that in the event of errors only the minimum amount of data would have to be re-entered.

In the light of these proposals modifications were made and included in the system which is now described.

Implementation with Graphics Tablet Input

It was decided that the best way to use the graphics tablet/pad was to imitate an audiogram such as that used in common clinical practice, by using an identical overlay on the touch-sensitive area. The philosophy here was that the clinician would complete the audiogram in the same manner as usually practised in the clinic, with the additional advantage that the hearing threshold levels would be automatically recorded and sent to the computer.

The important feature of this pad is that it enables the standard clinical audiogram card to be fitted in the touch-sensitive area. The implementation of this graphics tablet would then enable the input of hearing threshold levels directly as they are being recorded on the clinical audiogram card for the first time. This would combine the computer-based system with existing clinical practice with very little overhead in time. After entering the hearing threshold levels the clinician is automatically in possession of the traditionally adopted record audiograms and the computer analysed presentation simultaneously.

The standard clinical audiogram form used at Kent and Canterbury Hospital has three sets of audiograms as shown in Fig. 7.13. Each set consists of an audiogram for the left and right ears. It is common clinical practice at the hospital for patients to have their ears tested more than once during a course of treatment in order to monitor progress. An audiogram card such as that described above enables the results of these tests to be kept together for

AUDIOGRAM SHEET
KENT AND CANTERBURY HOSPITAL

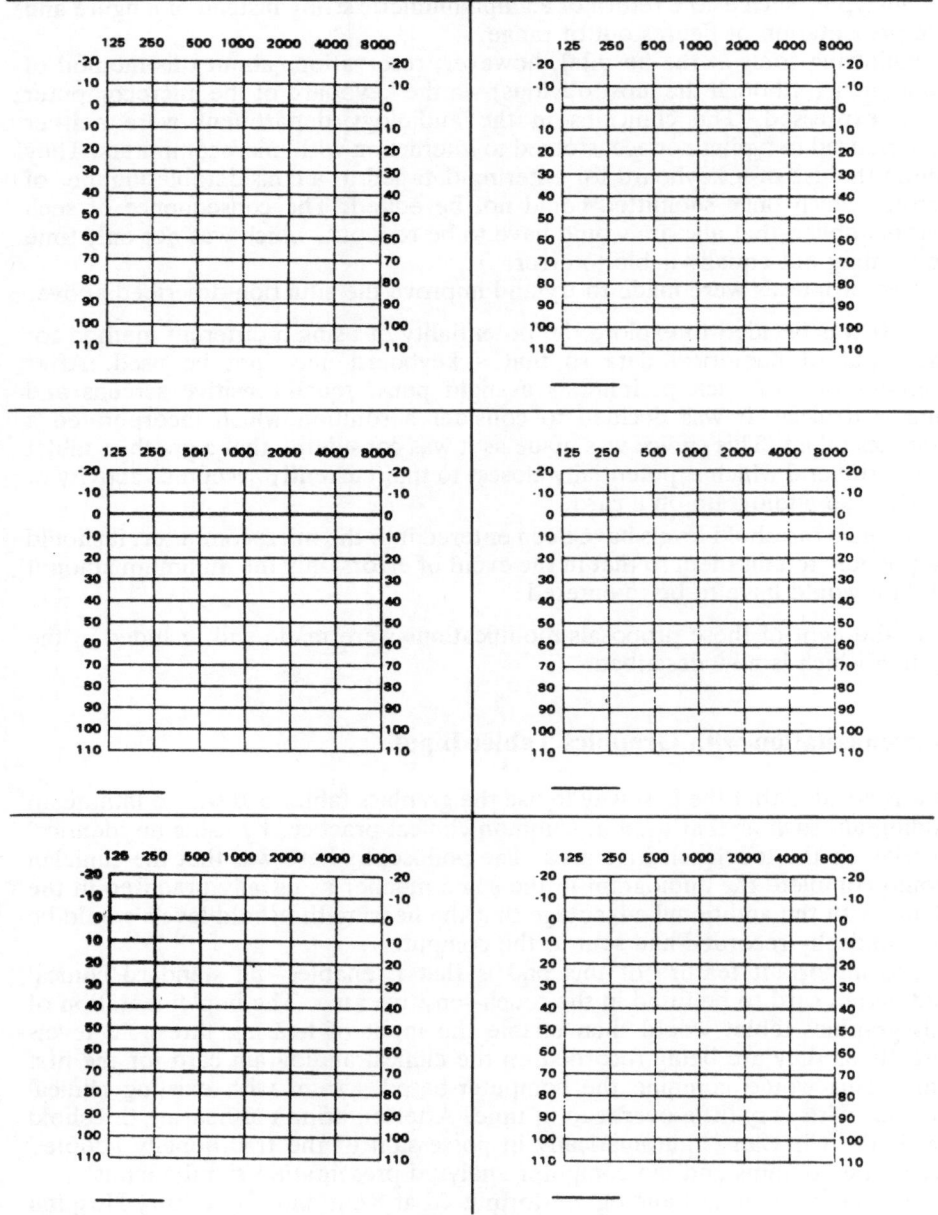

Fig. 7.13.   Standard clinical audiogram card used at Kent and Canterbury Hospital.

reference. It was decided that in incorporating the graphics tablet, the system should be made capable of recording all three sets of audiograms in a similar way, so that comparisons between them could again be made, even when the computer-based analysis was required.

Procedure

The standard clinical audiogram card (shown in Fig. 7.13) is placed on the touch-sensitive area of the pad. Initial data such as the patient's name, age and sex are input in the same manner as with the last system as use of the keyboard is by far the fastest method of acquiring this type of data in comparison to other commonly available peripherals. The following prompt is then issued.

Is touch pad to be used? (Y or N): Y

As with previous prompts of this type, if the returned string variable does not contain Y as its first character then the response is ignored and the prompt re-issued. Should the response to the above prompt be N, then the procedure for obtaining hearing threshold levels from the keyboard as described earlier will be adopted. If the response is positive (i.e. Y) then the screen is cleared and a plotting grid, in the form of an audiogram, is displayed as editing mode is entered.

The heading to the plotting grid makes it clear to the clinician which of the three audiograms he is completing. Information is also displayed which defines the ear to which the current entry of hearing threshold levels relates. The clinician can now proceed to plot the hearing thresholds on the conventional audiogram card, and each time a threshold level is plotted a circle or cross (depending on which ear is being plotted) marks the respective point on the plotting grid displayed on the monitor screen. This provides a valuable check that the computer has received the correct information on the intensity and frequency at which the hearing threshold level has been recorded. This facility also enables the clinician to see all the points that are currently recorded for that ear. Should any points need to be edited, subsequent points may be re-entered at any time. Only the last set of points to be entered on the audiogram are retained and displayed.

Once the clinician has completed editing points for an audiogram and wishes it to be displayed in the usual manner, he need only touch the border surrounding the required audiogram on the graphics tablet. The audiogram is then displayed with the normal band superimposed as illustrated earlier. Any audiogram on the card may be displayed in this manner allowing rapid comparisons to be made.

The commands controlling the system described earlier in this section are selected by touching the appropriate command from a menu at the top of the graphics tablet. The set of commands is somewhat reduced, however, as a result of the increased simplicity of the system. The remaining commands, Grid, Ext, Med, New and Help, however, all function in the same manner as described earlier.

System Assessment

A microcomputer-based system has been developed to display and analyse the hearing threshold levels resulting from a clinical hearing test. The display of the thresholds has been in the form of a graphical representation of a clinical audiogram displayed on the screen of a computer monitor which can be reproduced on paper using a printer. Analysis of the thresholds is made in two forms, the graphical superimposition of a normal band on the audiogram indicating the hearing threshold levels expected for a person of the stated age and sex, and the calculation of a figure of merit indicating the deviation of the patient's hearing levels from the accepted norm.

The numerical data required for the above analysis required some manipulation for them to be utilised appropriately on a microcomputer system, and finally a method of calculating the data from a set of mathematical equations was adopted. The method by which the hearing threshold levels of the patient were to be entered to the microcomputer required considerable investigation. After several clinical trials and experimentation involving numerous studies, it was decided to utilise a touch-sensitive graphics tablet which enabled the clinician to record thresholds on a clinical audiogram in a traditional manner which were simultaneously entered into the microcomputer system.

It is considered that the system summarised above has met the requirements described in this chapter in the following ways:

1. The implementation of a touch-sensitive graphics tablet as described above has been judged both by feedback from clinical trials and conclusions resulting from laboratory experiments [9] to have reduced the possibility of errors occurring in the manual transcription of audiograms.

2. It is also apparent in the feedback from clinical trials that the graphical representation of the clinical audiogram displayed by the system is a coherent representation of the patient's hearing threshold levels. It also provides more information than the conventional clinical audiogram in the form of patient data (name, age, and sex), numerically presented hearing threshold levels and analysis with respect to accepted normal values.

3. The system is very fast in calculating analytical data and presenting the audiogram graphically, and the method of the input of hearing thresholds (as described above) is no different from that performed in conventionally accepted clinical practice. It is also clear that the speed of response of the system does not conflict with current data entry procedures or operational practices.

As mentioned briefly above, there are two forms of analysis that are performed by the system, neither of which requires the experience of a departmental specialist. The first is the assessment of the effect of presbyacusis for a patient of specified age and sex, which is represented as a superimposed red normal band on the displayed audiogram. This gives an immediate indication of whether a patient's hearing is normal or not, depending on whether the line representing the hearing threshold levels is within the red band. The second form of analysis is the calculation of the deviation figure which gives an indication of how far below the accepted norm the patient's hearing response is considered to be.

The command structure which controls the system and the method of selecting these commands presented no problems to the clinical staff in the in situ trials.

In summary, the introduction of the microcomputer-based system into the Audiology Department of Kent and Canterbury Hospital has proved to be very successful. The clinical staff of the Department had little or no experience in operating computer-based systems before the current system was installed, and there are two main reasons why the system has been so well accepted and thought to be a valuable asset in clinical practice there.

1. The system is very easy to use since great care has been taken in the specification of the operator–system interface. It was a principal feature of the design that the user should have a minimum amount of data to enter and that data entry should be carried out in as clear and concise a manner as possible in order to be able to display the audiogram and acquire the required analysis. In this respect the system has proved successful as, in order to plot and display an audiogram, no extra interaction with the system is necessary than is required with the traditional method of transcription. The analysis performed by the system is achieved automatically without any need for a specific request or supervision from the user.

2. The microcomputer-based system is not intended to replace the present clinical system operated by the Audiology Department at the Hospital. The philosophy has always been to run the computer-based system in parallel with the traditional clinical system, ideally with the two systems merging into one.

Considering the points made above and the response from both clinical staff and the Departmental specialist at the Hospital, it is expected that the prototype system described will improve clinical practice in respect of both the efficiency in the recording of measurements and the information provided when the measurements are presented for analysis by the specialist. Fig. 7.14 shows a view

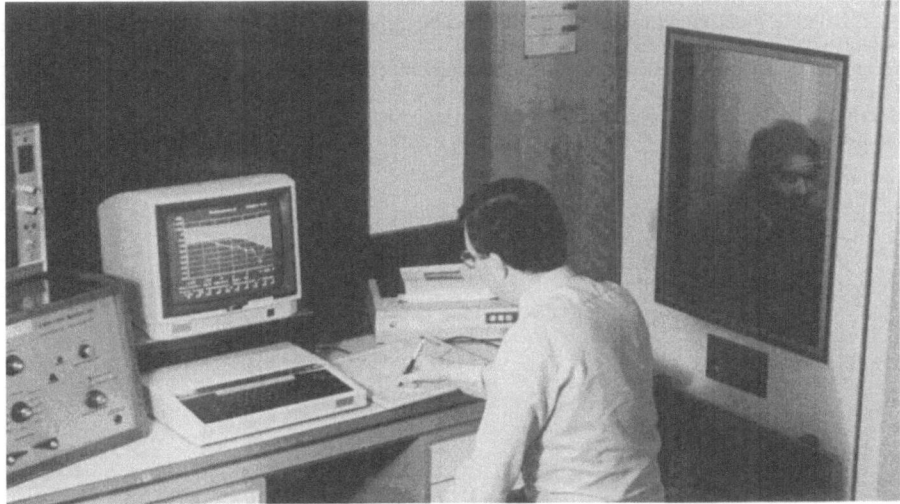

Fig. 7.14.   Photograph of prototype system in clinical use.

of the final prototype system. The microcomputer-based system described has been developed from original ideas and has not been based on any existing system. As far as it is known, no such application of microcomputers has been made in the analysis of hearing threshold levels in a clinical system before. This view is supported by discussions with a number of audiologists and industrial suppliers of audiology equipment who have shown interest in the system.

The research described here has led to the design and construction of a prototype microcomputer-based system for audiological testing. In moving towards the implementation stage, a number of very fundamental questions relating to data storage/access, data input/output, and man–machine interaction have been raised. The collaboration between Kent and Canterbury Hospital and the University of Kent has proved to be extremely fruitful, and has ensured that design decisions and system refinements have been based on sound and appropriate criteria. Longer-term trials will ultimately provide a final assessment of the value of the system, but the preliminary indications are that there is considerable scope for the introduction of computer-based technical aids in audiological practice.

References

1 Ginsberg IA, White TP (1978) In: Katz J (ed) Handbook of clinical audiology, chapter 2 Otological considerations in audiology. Williams & Wilkins, London, pp 9–10
2 Green DS (1978) In: Katz J (ed) Handbook of clinical audiology, chapter 9 Pure tone air-conduction testing. Williams & Wilkins, London, pp 105–108
3 International Organization for Standardization (1975) Acoustics – standard reference zero for the calibration of pure tone audiometers. International Standard ISO 389
4 Haughton PM (1980) Physical principles of audiology, chapter 5 Hearing disorders and the measurement of hearing. Adam Hilger, Bristol, pp 100–110
5 Ginsberg IA, White TP (1978) In: Katz J (ed) Handbook of clinical audiology, chapter 2 Otological considerations in audiology. Williams & Wilkins, London, pp 19–20
6 Robinson DW, Sutton GJ (1976) A comparative analysis of data on the relation of pure-tone audiometric thresholds to age. National Physical Laboratory Acoustics Report AC 84
7 Haughton PM (1980) Physical principles of audiology, chapter 7 Physical characteristics of speech. Adam Hilger, Bristol, pp 152–156
8 Health and Safety Executive Discussion Document (1978) Audiometry in industry. HMSO, London
9 Smith SL (1986) A microcomputer-assisted analysis of audiological test data in a clinical environment. MSc thesis, University of Kent at Canterbury

8 A Microcomputer-Based System for the Assessment of Postoperative Fatigue

S. Stock

Introduction

The use of a microcomputer to measure postoperative fatigue may seem to be a rather unusual application and therefore it is necessary to describe the background to the study and something of the thinking that was behind the project.

Postoperative fatigue is an ill-understood syndrome that is said to affect as many as 30 % of patients undergoing elective abdominal surgery. It is, however, one of those problems that seems to have been largely ignored by research workers and clinicians alike. This in itself is somewhat surprising in view of the fact that patients have been undergoing operations for so many years and one of the reasons is undoubtedly the difficulty in measuring fatigue in an objective manner. Another is the reluctance of many patients to bother their doctors with what they may feel is an expected part of their convalescence. Whether fatigue is to be expected and if so for how long it would normally last are two of the questions studied by Moss, Dohan and others in the 1950s [1]. A series of papers was written on various aspects of surgical convalescence and the findings were reported in the *Annals of the New York Academy of Sciences*. These include studies on psychological, social and economic factors as well as on medical ones. Although they relate to Americans in the 1950s and may therefore not be universally applicable they bring out some interesting points [1,2]. In particular no financial or social factors that influenced the duration of surgical convalescence were identified. However, Moss and Dohan noticed that a significant proportion of their patients experienced a period of fatigue which was especially marked in the first week or two after their return to work. In their summary, they discuss this finding:

Most individuals experience increased fatigue during the first week after their return to work. This readjustment period exists apparently without relation to the length of convalescence. What is the nature of the fatigue noticed by patients? Would it have occurred if the patient had not undergone surgery, but had simply been told by an authority figure that he must "take it easy"? Would he then have had the same degree of fatigue during the period of inactivity and on return to work? Is this period comparable to a training period of athletics? Would such fatigue have occurred had the patient increased his home activities even more? Is it associated with some metabolic or chemical change that we are not accustomed to measuring? These are some of the pertinent questions that remain unanswered.

In 1978 Rose and King reviewed the subject [3]. The conclusions they came to after extensively studying the available medical literature were as follows:

1. Performance characteristics of the central nervous, cardiovascular, respiratory and muscular systems postoperatively have received little investigative attention

2. A better understanding of the syndrome of postoperative fatigue could be achieved by a descriptive analysis of physiological performance postoperatively

The following year there was an Editorial in the *Lancet* [4] on the subject which stated: "Until postoperative fatigue has been properly defined and better ways are found to measure it, our almost total ignorance of this important matter will continue to be a trial to surgical patients and a nagging concern to their doctors."

Since that time the only published work on the subject has been from Denmark. Christensen and his co-workers studied the cardiovascular responses of surgical patients to sub-maximal exercise tests using a cycle ergometer postoperatively. They also used a linear analogue scale as a method of assessing the subjective feelings of fatigue [5] and, based on a change in their preoperative scores, defined two groups of patients following elective abdominal surgery. Those with an increase in the "fatigue score" of three or more units at one month postoperatively they called the "fatigued" group. This group comprised approximately one-third of the patients studied. Some evidence was put forward for a correlation between the feelings of fatigue and an increased pulse rate found during an orthostatic stress test. However the latter result needs to be interpreted with caution. In their second paper [6], again using the linear analogue scale, Christensen and his co-workers produced some evidence to suggest that catabolic changes such as loss in body weight and triceps skinfold thickness in the peri-operative period were more marked in the fatigued patients.

There has been some research performed which has a bearing on the subject of postoperative fatigue although it is not directly related to it; Wood [7] studied postoperative exercise capacity in surgical patients using a bicycle ergometer and found that it was reduced by 20%–25%. He attributed this to a change in the work capacity of large muscle masses. However, no attempt was made to measure changes in muscle mass. Edwards et al. [8] studied postoperative changes in muscle function and found that isokinetic endurance was reduced in almost all of their patients for at least 3 weeks and in some cases as much as 5 weeks. Arnold et al. [9] described a patient suffering from a post-viral fatigue syndrome in whom they found excessive intracellular acidosis of skeletal muscle on exercise.

Thus it will be seen that there exists a great need for an objective method of assessing fatigue in order to allow more specific and accurate documentation of the syndrome to be undertaken.

What Is Fatigue?

Fatigue was first studied in depth in relation to muscle function by Waller in the late nineteenth century [10,11]. He also studied the problem of whether it was perceived centrally or peripherally. Since then a great deal of work has been carried out on muscles in vitro and in vivo in an attempt to define the underlying physiological basis for the phenomenon. As yet there are no clear conclusions to be drawn from these studies although suggested factors in the pathophysiology include:

1. A depressed activity in rate determining glycolytic enzymes, notably phosphofructokinase [12]
2. Reduced numbers of type 2 muscle fibres [13]
3. Reduced intracellular potassium and water [14]

On the other hand, little work has been undertaken concerning the whole individual.

Fatigue consists of three components: weakness; an increased awareness of the effort required to perform a task; a sensation present in muscles even when they are not being used.

Attempts to measure fatigue have usually concentrated on the first of these as it is the easiest to measure. As far as subjective assessment is concerned some sort of rating scale is necessary. The only two applicable ones to date have been the linear analogue scale of Christensen which is quite likely to give non-uniform results [15] and the *Rating of Perceived Exertion* scale devised by Borg [16]. The latter has been used mostly in conjunction with exercise tests.

There are several methods available for the assessment of a patient's physical performance:

1. Maximal voluntary muscle contraction [17]
2. Grip strength [18]
3. Isokinetic endurance [7]
4. Oxygen uptake [19]

All these methods however suffer from drawbacks. The first three are all assessments made on either an individual muscle or a group of muscles and therefore have a somewhat limited applicability. They mostly require strict laboratory conditions for their use, and use bulky and non-portable equipment. It was for these reasons that they were felt to be unsuitable for a study of postoperative fatigue.

The Measurement of Activity

In order to test the hypothesis that if a patient feels fatigued then he will be less active we have sought to find a way of measuring activity. If the hypothesis proves to be true then we will have an indirect but objective way of measuring fatigue.

Activity can be subdivided into three components in much the same way as metabolic rate. This is not surprising as the two are closely related.

1. Baseline activity i.e. sleeping
2. Activity of daily living e.g. sitting, eating, walking
3. Recreational activity e.g. sport

Activity is characterised qualitatively by two dominant features, posture and movement. In addition, a quantitative measurement would include an assessment of cardiac output and muscle work. Unfortunately it is not yet feasible to obtain an absolute measure of a person's activity over an extended period; ideally we would like to be able to measure the total oxygen consumption which would allow an overall measure of metabolic rate to be obtained. However, there are ways in which some progress can be made towards this ideal and these will be discussed later. It is not essential to have an absolute measure as a relative one is suitable for comparing performance by the same patient on several different occasions. Thus, provided methods are standardised as far as possible, it should be feasible to obtain meaningful and reproducible results.

An important consideration when studying a person's activity is that the method used for recording should interfere as little as possible with that activity. In this context it means that their normal daily routine should not be upset. Various methods exist as listed below:

1. Diary. The patient is asked to keep a diary of his activities. This method requires a high level of motivation from the patient and suffers from a considerable degree of inaccuracy
2. Time and Motion Study. This method is very labour-intensive and is not suitable for use over long periods or in the patient's home
3. Assisted Recall. Various indirect time and motion methods have been tried. These reduce the problems associated with a diary method but still depend on the patient's ability to recall events accurately. However they offer considerable advantages over the above methods [20]
4. Video Recording. This is mainly of use for comparing people in groups and would not be applicable to the domiciliary environment

Ambulatory Monitoring

Ambulatory monitoring has been used for many years in a variety of different ways. For example, electroencephalogram recording, oesophageal pH monitoring and even the measurement of muscle tremor. Its widest use however has undoubtedly been for electrocardiogram monitoring where it is particularly useful in the assessment of patients with transient arrhythmias or syncopal attacks. The system we have been using is based on one developed in Glasgow [21]. It was initially used there to monitor performance of amputees using different types of artificial limbs. It has several advantages over the methods listed above for this type of study. These are:

1. It is comfortable and unobtrusive and therefore interferes little with the patients' activity
2. It is not dependent upon the patients' ability to recall events accurately. However it may be complemented by the use of a diary if required in order to provide greater detail
3. Multiple physiological parameters may be recorded simultaneously. The system we have developed measures the following parameters: posture i.e. lying, sitting or standing; body movement; electrocardiogram; elapsed time; "Events" as noted by the patient

From these data we are able to derive further information as described below.

Method

The equipment used is based around an Oxford Medical Systems four-track tape recorder (Medilog). This device records four channels of analogue data onto a standard width cassette tape. The tape runs at 2 mm/second to allow a recording time of 24 hours with a C-120 cassette. This reduces the bandwidth of signals that may be recorded to 100 Hertz but this is adequate for the present uses. The recorder is powered by four mercury batteries which provide a voltage of 5.4 volts. These have a life-time of approximately 36 hours in continuous use. They are non-rechargeable as unfortunately there are no currently available rechargeable batteries with sufficient capacity to allow an uninterrupted 24-hour recording to be made whilst keeping the unit self-contained. The apparatus weighs approximately 400 g.

The sensors themselves are of three types and are attached to the patient's chest and leg with tape. The leads pass under the clothes to make the system less noticeable. The three types of electrode will be described in turn.

Electrocardiograph Electrode. These are standard disposable electrodes (3M Red Dot) although non-disposable ones are equally satisfactory. The main concern is to obtain a clear signal that is free from artefacts due to factors such as body and clothing movement. This is achieved by attention to certain details:

1. Scrupulous cleaning and preparation of the patient's skin using isopropyl alcohol and then fine emery paper and shaving where necessary. This has the effect of reducing the contact resistance
2. Secure anchoring of the leads to prevent them from pulling on the electrodes
3. The choice of sites for attachment that are not covered with too much mobile subcutaneous fat. In practice the best sites are often over the sternum and the left lower ribs in the mid-axillary line. The exact positions are not critical as a standard lead pattern is not necessary for the subsequent analysis. Despite

following the above steps it may still be difficult to obtain a clean signal in certain obese patients, especially if they are fairly active

Accelerometers. The first accelerometers used were ones that were marketed by Oxford Medical Systems. However, although they functioned well at first, they proved to be somewhat fragile after extended use and as they have now been discontinued it has been necessary to design our own. These were made by our medical physics department and are based on the piezo-electric principle. They consist of a small crystal (from a record player cartridge) to which a small weight is attached by means of a flexible metal strip (the stylus). When the sensor moves (i.e. accelerates) the crystal is deformed as the weight lags behind. This produces an electrical signal which is amplified and recorded onto the tape. The whole is enclosed in silicone rubber for the comfort of the patient and is approximately $1 \times 2.5 \times 0.5$ cm in size. The sensor is placed over the patient's sternum in such a way as to detect the vertical oscillations that occur during the stance and swing phases of walking. The accelerometer is much more sensitive to acceleration in one plane than others and this is indicated on the sensor to ensure correct positioning. The waveform approximates to a sine wave under these circumstances. The mass of the weight in the sensor is important as it governs the frequency response of the sensor and the degree of damping it exhibits; thus if the mass is too great the sensor will not respond properly to higher frequencies and if it is too small it will vibrate excessively and produce artefacts.

There are, of course, other ways of detecting walking and one of the most successful is the use of a footfall detector such as a thin-film capacitance transducer [22,23]. This device is worn as part of the sole of a shoe under the foot and the capacitance varies with the weight of the patient compressing it. This can be used to produce a varying voltage output in the same way as our original design of posture sensors (see below). The disadvantage of this type of device is firstly that it is subjected to considerable wear and tear, secondly that it is not really suitable for monitoring over long periods and thirdly that there needs to be a long wire attached to the patient's leg which may reduce the acceptability of the device to the wearer.

Posture Sensors. There are many approaches to the design of what is effectively a gravity detector. The first design we used consisted of a circular non-conductive tube surrounded by wire braiding containing a small quantity of mercury. As the sensor was tipped it changed its capacitance and, in conjunction with an oscillator, this was used to produce an offset voltage. This signal was then recorded onto the tape. The advantage of this system was that it gave a measure of the angle from vertical of the sensor. The disadvantage was that it only operated in one plane. Other designs are available which produce similar information such as optical systems which use a variable density filter between the light source and the detector, but they suffer from the same drawback.

The second design uses gravity switches. These produce a stepped output with discrete voltages for each posture and this has proved to be an advantage for our use. In addition they operate in all planes. They consist of a small chamber filled with inert gas containing two electrodes and a small quantity of mercury. The inert gas prevents oxidation of the mercury which would otherwise result in unreliable switching. When the sensor is tipped the mercury which normally bridges the gap between the electrodes uncovers one of them and opens the circuit. Two of these sensors are used, one placed over the patient's sternum and the other on the thigh. When the patient is standing both switches are closed. If the patient sits down, the switch on the leg opens and if the patient lies down they are both open. The sensors are connected to a constant-current generator and the changing resistance produces a corresponding change in the output voltage which is recorded onto the tape.

The switches should ideally switch at an angle of 45 degrees from the vertical in any plane as this produces the best discrimination between postures. (People rarely sit bolt upright in chairs or lie completely flat in bed.) In actual fact there is considerable variation between the switches and it is necessary to select appropriate ones. The precise switching angle varies between planes and so they must be orientated correctly. The other problem with the devices is that they exhibit hysteresis, in other words there is an angle between the position for a clean on signal and that for a clean off signal. In practice however this is only of the order of 5 degrees and does not seem to produce any artefacts. These sensors have been widely tested both in the laboratory and on patients and have proved to be very reliable. Once again they are encased in silicone rubber which has the additional advantage of preventing the leads from being pulled off.

The recordings are usually made while the patient is at home and the equipment is fitted after it has been carefully explained and demonstrated to the patient. Failure to do this can result in some quite alarming misconceptions. (One patient, for example, was worried that his speech was going to be recorded throughout the 24 hours!). The patient is asked to keep a diary of any particular changes in activity if possible. Examples would be going out for a walk, going to bed or relaxing in front of the television. At these times he presses the "event button" on the recorder. This superimposes a signal on the timing channel of the recorder which lasts for 13 seconds and can be detected separately from the clock pulses derived from the in-built oscillator. Although this information was of great assistance in the interpretation of the recordings early in the study it is now used much less. After completion of the 24-hour recording period, during which the patient carries out his normal daily activities, he is again visited at home and the equipment removed. There have been very few problems associated with the use of the equipment although a few patients appear to become allergic to the tape used to affix the sensors. This has not caused anything more than slight irritation in the majority of cases and is avoided by changing the type of tape used during subsequent recordings.

At the start of the study the tapes were replayed using the Oxford Medical Systems PB 2 replay unit and the output recorded onto a four-channel chart recorder (Fig. 8.1). The playback unit replays all four channels of data simultaneously at high speed (12 cm/second) which takes 24 minutes. It provides amplified outputs for analysis and displays time which can be derived from the tape signal. This takes the form of either elapsed time since the start of the recording in hours and minutes or time on a 24-hour clock. This is especially useful for pinpointing particular events or periods of interest and can be combined with the patient's diary for interpretation of the data. However, it quickly became obvious that the interpretation of the resulting chart output would be at best time-consuming and tedious and at worst impossible and it was for this reason that it was decided to adopt a microcomputer-based system to perform the analysis of the tapes (Fig. 8.2).

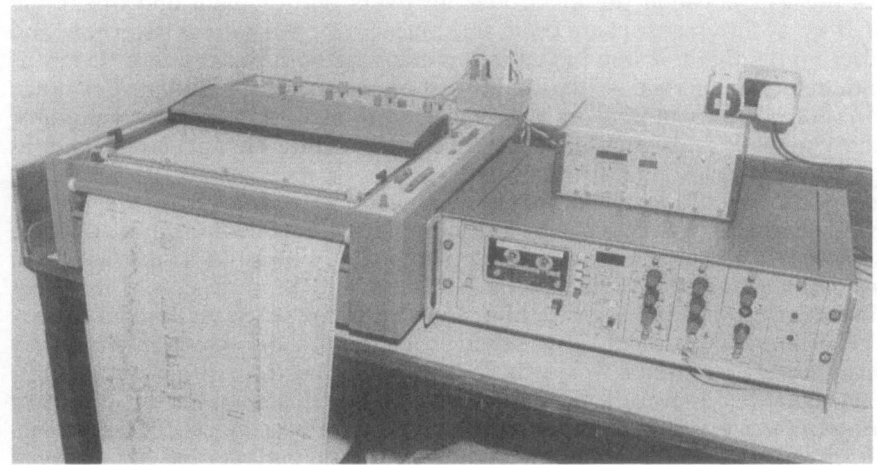

Fig. 8.1. Original tape replay system.

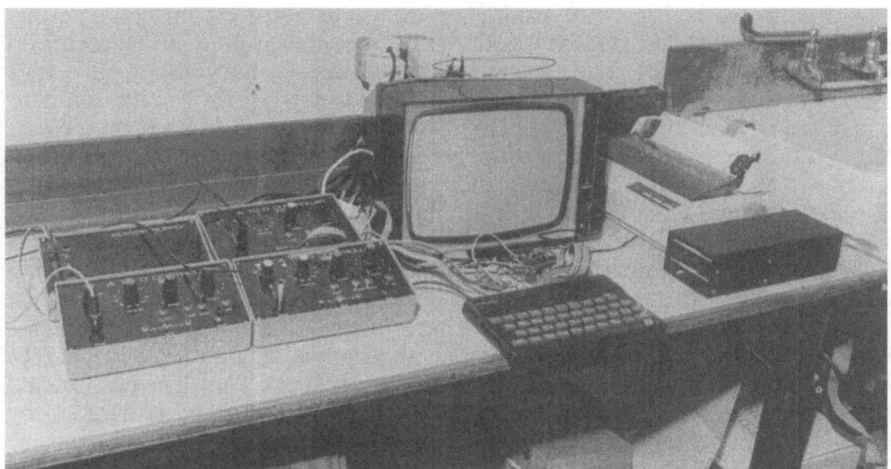

Fig. 8.2. Microcomputer based tape analysis system.

Data Processing

An ideal data processing system should have the following features:

1. It should be flexible enough to follow changes in the direction of the research
2. It should allow the whole tape to be analysed in a single pass
3. It should not be expensive to produce or maintain

4. It should produce accurate and reproducible results in an easily interpreted format
5. It should be user-friendly

Although our system does not yet fulfil all of these criteria (in particular it is not user-friendly) it can be upgraded to do so when time allows and when the need arises.

From the raw data recorded on the tape in analogue form, certain information is required: elapsed time; mean heart rate; mean heart rate by posture; number of steps walked. We can consider each of these in turn.

Elapsed Time. Although the capstan speed of the recorders is carefully controlled there are variations in tape speed due to such things as stretching of the tape (this is a problem only with the thinner tape of C-120 cassettes) and external pressure on the recorder from its being sat on! Therefore, in order accurately to record elapsed time, a signal is recorded onto one channel of the tape at the time of the recording of other data and this is subsequently used as a reference for the analysis program.

Mean Heart Rate. The signal recorded onto the tape is an electrocardiographic trace. This is useful for cardiologists and those involved with the investigation of rhythm disorders but it is of no relevance to the present study. To obtain the heart rate the QRS complexes are counted and then expressed as beats per minute. This value can be averaged over a whole hour or any other period of time.

Mean Heart Rate by Posture. There is evidence from experimental studies [5,24,25] that the heart-rate response to exercise following bed rest or surgery is altered. Whether this is due to resetting of the basal heart rate or because a greater circulatory load exists for a given level of exertion is not certain. By producing an overall average heart rate for each posture it is hoped to provide further insight into this phenomenon. In other words, the analysis produces an average heart rate for the whole time that the patient was sitting during the 24 hours of the recording, and corresponding values for lying and standing.

Number of Steps Walked. The output is expressed as the number of steps taken per hour for each hour of the day. As the tape is replayed at high speed, it is not possible to reproduce the output from the accelerometer channel onto a chart recorder to produce a meaningful trace. The frequency of the signal is of the order of 50–100 Hz. Because of the problems associated with obtaining this sort of data manually an analogue to digital converter was designed to allow the analogue tape signals to be fed into the microcomputer. The initial system was constructed to assess the practicability of the project and also to try to identify any particular problems that might hamper the development of a more complex system. It consists of a dual-channel analogue to digital converter (ADC). The accelerometer channel was chosen for the prototype as it was easy to standardise the output for calibration purposes.

The microcomputer chosen was a Sinclair Spectrum with 48 K RAM. There were three reasons: availability, working knowledge of Z-80 machine code and interfacing components were easily obtainable.

Hardware

An 8-bit successive approximation ADC was chosen. This allows 256 discrete levels to be detected, which does not compare favourably with the 4096 steps of a 12-bit device but is sufficient for this purpose. In addition, interfacing is very much simpler with the 8-bit device. It was achieved via an 8255 programmable peripheral interface (Fig. 8.3). It has three ports which can be software selected as input, output or a combination of both. One port is used as an input to receive data from the ADC and the others as outputs to control switching of the signal inputs. The input was routed via a sample and hold circuit which reduces errors from rapidly changing signals by freezing the input voltage while the analogue to digital conversion takes place. This is more important when high-frequency signals are being analysed and is a refinement which may not be strictly necessary. A variable gain amplifier/attenuator was used to increase the range of signals that were suitable for analysis. This allowed inputs of between 50 mV and 20 V to produce a full output from the ADC. Therefore the corresponding voltage changes required to be detected by the ADC are of the order of 195 uV to 78 mV. The ADC used allows a maximum sampling rate of 30 kHz. The system is powered from its own power supply, there not being any spare capacity available from the computer's power supply (Fig. 8.2). The second channel was used for the timing signals from the tape so that these could be used to control the program timing.

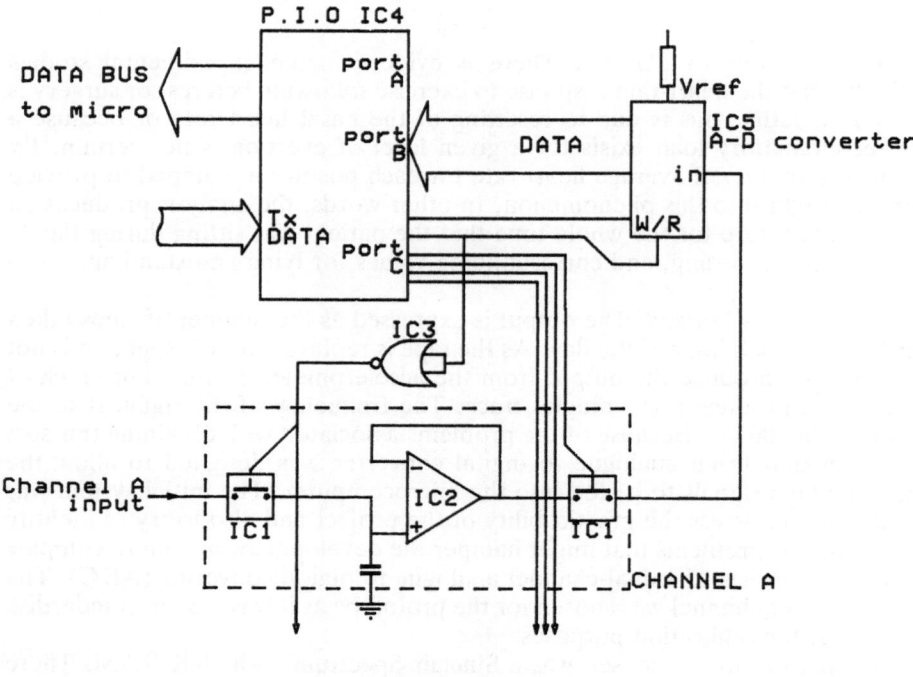

Fig. 8.3. Analogue to digital converter interface.

Software

During initial testing of the system a commercially available program (Digiscope 3–Digisound Ltd.) was utilised. This program allows the Spectrum to be used as a digital storage oscilloscope which was of assistance in studying the input waveforms and amplitudes of tape-derived signals. Once expertise had been gained it was no longer necessary to use it. It was necessary to write a program for the tape analysis. An initial program was written in BASIC but this was too slow for this application with a maximum sampling rate for signals of 18 Hz. It was adequate for the timing signals but not for the accelerometer (or electrocardiograph) channel.

It is accepted that in order to avoid output distortion from an effect known as aliasing (which is caused by interaction between the input signal and the ADC clock frequency) the input should not contain any significant harmonics of frequency greater than half the sampling rate. We then wrote the program in machine code and the opposite problem occurred as the program ran at a clock frequency greater than the maximum sampling rate of the ADC. All these frequencies are an order of magnitude greater than required for sampling the accelerometer signal and so it was necessary to introduce delays in the program to slow it down (see below). The arithmetic manipulations performed were within the capabilities of the Spectrum.

The Program

No attempt was made to make the initial program user friendly as it was a temporary system by one of the authors. The data from the ADC is passed via the programmable peripheral interface as 8-bit binary numbers to the input ports of the microcomputer. These can be read easily by the use of a single command in either BASIC or machine code and stored in a register for subsequent manipulation. In addition to the accelerometer channel, timing was taken from the tape to synchronise the counting and allow division of the overall count into hourly aliquots. This gives a result for the number of steps walked during each hour of the day.

At this stage a variety of test procedures were employed to test the system. It was straightforward to check that the timing part of the program was functioning as the playback monitor's display of elapsed time could be used for reference. No problems were encountered with this. The part of the program dealing with the accelerometer channel which is a pulse counter was tested initially using a sine-wave generator. The next stage was to record a known number of steps onto the tape and replay this. It soon became clear that the counting of regular waveforms such as a pure sine wave did not present any problems, but that the signal from the accelerometer was anything but pure, containing a variety of artefacts. The most prominent of these was found to be a high-frequency spike that was superimposed on the main sinusoidal waveform. This was found to be attributable to the heel strike phase of walking where the impact of the person's foot hitting the ground was detected by the accelerometer as a short-lived deceleration phase. A number of solutions were tried including cushioning the accelerometer with foam rubber but they were not very successful. As the artefacts were mostly high frequency relative to the walking signal it was possible to filter them out using a fairly sharp cut-off low pass filter (24 dB/octave). Once again the digital oscilloscope program was of help in selecting the optimum settings for this. The waveform became nearer to a sine wave although at a somewhat reduced amplitude. We could have reduced the problem of interference by damping the sensor more heavily either mechanically or electrically, but this was not thought to be necessary. Another problem that was encountered was that of body movement detected while the person was travelling in a car. The source of movement was from uneven road surfaces rather than acceleration and braking as the position of the sensor on the chest largely eliminated the detection of acceleration in an antero-posterior plane. Studies on the power spectra of motor vehicle vibration [26] show that the range of frequencies of vertical acceleration expected overlaps that of slow walking (i.e. around 1 Hz). This type of artefact is therefore not amenable to filtering and there did not appear to be any satisfactory solution to the problem other than obtaining details of the times of journeys from the patient. In the Mark II system a change in program design has allowed this to be dealt with. Interestingly, recordings on a patient who was working as a train driver did not show the same effect and so this does not seem to be a problem with rail travel. Although considerable problems had been experienced with the accelerometer channel, the others have been relatively free of noise and artefacts and therefore they have not been so difficult to incorporate into the Mark II system.

The other important factor was found to be the precise method used for detecting a pulse by the microcomputer. The use of a decision based solely on whether the input level exceeds a pre-determined reference level was found to be inadequate as over-counting occurred. Further details on the method used are described below in the section on the program in current use.

Mark II Hardware

Once the prototype system was working it was modified to fulfil the requirements of the study. The block diagram of the system is shown in Fig. 8.4. The first change made was to increase the number of input channels on the ADC

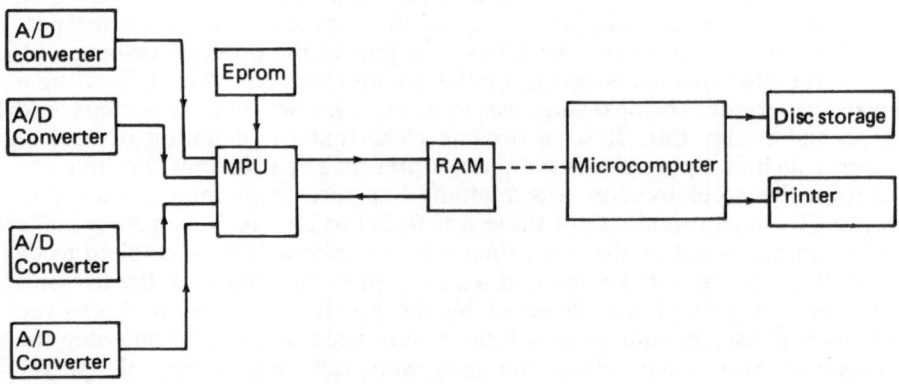

Fig. 8.4. Digital recording and processing system.

to four. To do this required the use of a rudimentary multiplexing system to select the inputs as only one could be read by the ADC at a time. This was achieved using analogue switches (Fig. 8.3). These devices are controlled by Port C of the programmable peripheral interface (IC.4) and can therefore be controlled in turn by the software. The two analogue switches in IC.1 (Fig. 8.3) are connected to both the input and output of the sample and hold circuit (IC.2).

The switches for all channels, except the one to be read, are set open-circuit. Before conversion takes place, the switches on both input and output of IC.2 are closed. The one on the input only remains closed momentarily while the input voltage is stored in the capacitor. The switch on the output remains closed until it has been read and converted. In this way rapid switching between inputs can be achieved.

Preliminary processing of the electrocardiograph channel was already available in the form of an integrator which provided a continuous read-out of the average heart rate in beats per minute. By using this instead of the ECG signal the programming was simplified and the need for a filter obviated as the resulting signal is a DC voltage. Hence in Fig. 8.5 only three filters are shown. An additional benefit was that a variable gain amplifier was not necessary for this channel, thus reducing the bulk of the hardware. The other channels have been provided with variable gain amplifiers to increase the flexibility of the system and allow optimal settings for signal levels to be selected throughout.

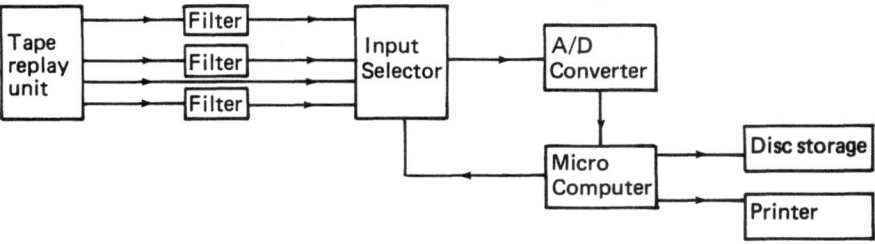

Fig. 8.5.   Automatic data processing system Mark II.

Although many early problems had been experienced with the accelerometer channel the others have been relatively free of noise and artefacts and therefore have not been difficult to incorporate into the Mark II system.

The Program (Mark II)

The simplified algorithm for the machine code section of the program is shown in Fig. 8.6. The hardware is initialised by defining the ports on the programmable peripheral interface (PPI). The posture channel is next sampled, and then the heart rate, which is added to the relevant stores. (There is one for calculation of mean heart rate and one each for lying, sitting and standing.) If the patient is found to be standing then the accelerometer channel is sampled, otherwise it is ignored. In this way the majority of the artefacts discussed above can be eliminated. The timing channel is then sampled and if an hour has elapsed (recorded time) then the necessary calculations are performed and the values stored. The cycle then re-starts and continues until the time is completed. Once

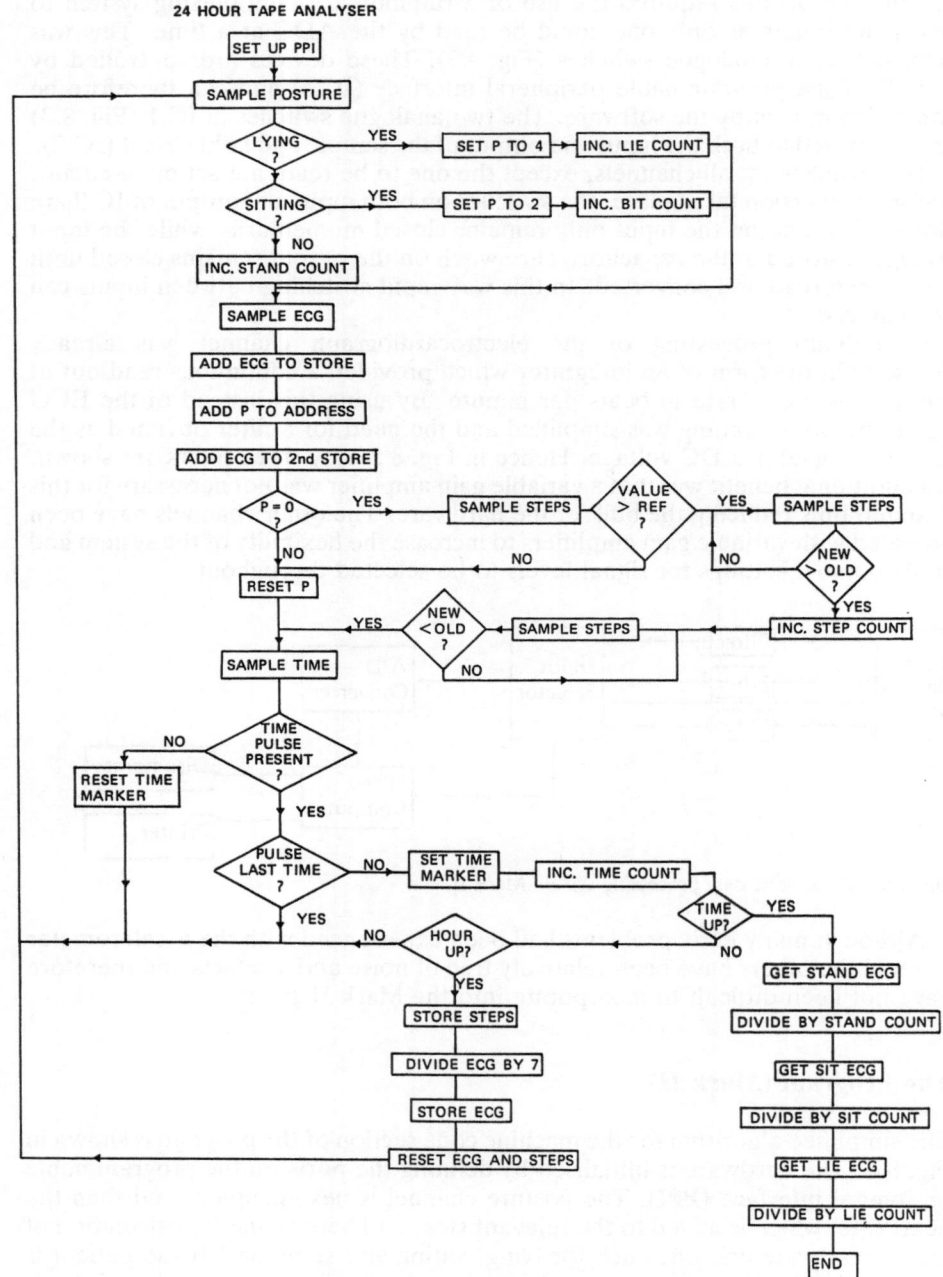

Fig. 8.6. Algorithm for 24-hour tape analyser. PPI, programmable peripheral interface; INC, increment (increase by 1); P, a variable used for indexed addressing.

the accelerometer channel is sampled several criteria need to be met before a step is counted, to reduce mis-counting from artefacts and noise.

1. The input must exceed a pre-determined reference level
2. There must be a detectable up-slope to the waveform
3. The up-slope must be followed by a detectable down-slope

For the sake of clarity the algorithm has been drawn without any delay loops. These are necessary because of the high speed at which machine code is executed. By way of example, in the accelerometer channel sampling routine, a gradually increasing input voltage is tested for several times successively before an up-slope to the waveform is registered and the next step is executed. At normal running speed, assuming an input voltage of half the maximum in the form of a regular waveform such as a triangular one, a frequency of less than approximately 100 Hz would not be changing rapidly enough to fulfil the criteria for an up-slope. Therefore, since this sort of frequency range is being measured, the program has to be slowed down considerably to cater for it. Similar considerations apply in other parts of the program.

Once the tape has finished, the final values are calculated and stored, then the program returns to BASIC. Various options are available to print the results on the screen or printer in the form of a simple list, histogram (Fig. 8.7) or a "circle-gram". The former displays the number of steps taken each hour and mean heart rate for each hour, the latter either one or the other. Results can also be stored on 3½-inch floppy discs for future reference. One of the disadvantages of using the Sinclair Spectrum is that it is not IBM-compatible and so the results cannot easily be downloaded onto a main-frame computer for analysis.

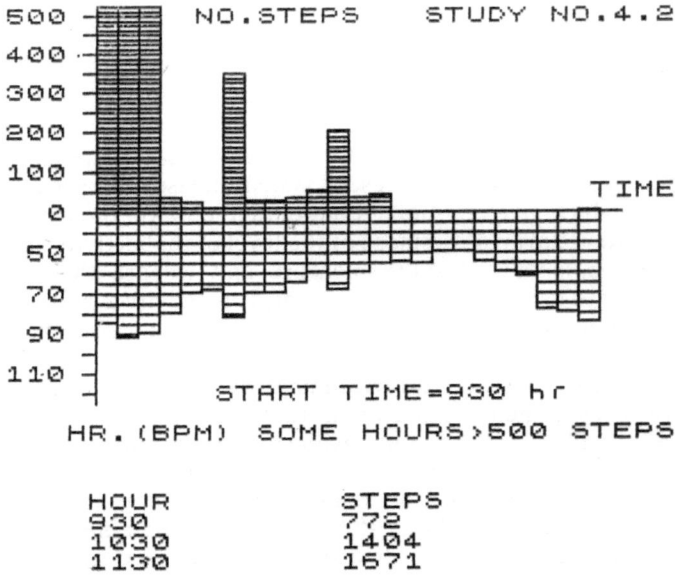

Fig. 8.7. Example of a microcomputer printed output.

Nevertheless, the more straightforward statistics can be performed on the Spectrum and the use of random access files makes this quite convenient.

The System in Use

At the start of each analysis session the equipment is calibrated. This consists of several steps but only takes a few minutes to do:

1. The output of the ADC is checked to ensure that zero volts on each input produces an output of 127/128 (the response of the ADC is bipolar in this configuration). This is done by a subroutine in the BASIC program.

2. The chart recorder calibration is checked. This is still used alongside the computer as it provides a quick way of scanning for artefacts such as disconnection of a lead from an ECG electrode. The microcomputer will not detect these. The chart recorder displays heart rate, posture and an indication of body movement as well as elapsed time. Its main use is to check that the various sensors are working correctly as from time to time loose connections do develop or sensors get pulled out of position by active patients. These problems give erroneous results that are easy to spot on the chart output.

3. Once a week the input levels of the signals are checked using the oscilloscope program to ensure that they are of the right magnitude.

4. Each tape is replayed and may be left unattended. The chart output is inspected and the results of the analysis stored. The whole process takes approximately 30 minutes.

Future Development

Ideally we would like to be able to measure the total energy expenditure by the patient for the whole 24-hour period. The present system measures a series of physiological parameters which give additional quantitative data on the activity of the person allowing us to make an assessment of the level of that activity. This is still a long way from being an absolute measure and we are therefore investigating different ways to try to improve it. In studies on activity a confusing variety of indices has been described and used; most of these use measurements of the heart rate, for example time spent with a heart rate of >50 % of the total reserve or the time spent with a heart rate exceeding that of steady walking. These are also relative measurements, but Rodahl [27] tried to get round this problem. He obtained graphs of heart rate against oxygen uptake during submaximal exercise testing on a bicycle ergometer. He then used the heart rate to predict the oxygen uptake of the same individuals engaged in other activities. Using this system he obtained results within ±15 % of the value obtained by the Douglas-bag technique. He concluded ". . . the use of recorded heart rate in the field . . . may be used as a basis for the estimation of work load when the same, large muscle groups are used as in the bicycle work". The main problem encountered in the patients we are studying is that they often have energy expenditures that are near base-line levels. This is because they may feel unwell preoperatively as a result of their underlying pathology, they may experience pain postoperatively, they may experience postoperative fatigue, and some of them are old and may not be very active even when well.

At these low levels of exercise, the oxygen uptake/heart rate relationship is weaker because psychological and other factors play a large part in determining the heart rate as it approaches the resting level. This method may allow us to calculate the overall oxygen uptake more realistically than before.

An alternative approach is to use calculated figures for the energy expenditure of certain activities. Several studies have looked closely at this subject. One by Fox et al. [28] coins the term METS for Multiples of the Metabolic Needs for Sitting Quietly and another [29] quotes absolute figures based on the authors' own studies. Using these figures it is possible to obtain an estimated figure for the overall energy expenditure above basal level based on the data obtained from the ambulatory monitoring. Both these former approaches assume that the oxygen uptake/heart rate relationship is not altered after surgery. Although few data are available on this subject the work of Christensen [5] would appear to support this hypothesis.

Digital Recording

The system described above has overcome many problems related to the interpretation of data from the ambulatory monitoring system and it has made it practical to use in this way. It does not avoid the need for a recording tape and this is the weak point in the system. The tape records analogue data and although this is essential for certain applications such as ECG and EEG recording it is not for this one. In fact, it has been estimated that a 24-hour tape can hold many megabytes of data whereas, using the above system, we reduce this to a little over 100 bytes. Therefore less than 0.01 % of the original data is retained! It would make sense to use a digital recording system with on-line data processing to reduce this overkill. Such a system has several advantages over a conventional analogue system:

1. There are no moving parts. This eliminates problems of a mechanical nature which are encountered with the tape recorders, including variable tape speed, tape jamming and mechanical wear. The tape recorders make a persistent whirring sound when running and although this is not particularly loud, some patients find it distracting. The recorder can also be subjected to more extreme environments if there are no moving parts and this is very useful when monitoring people at work. The tapes used by the conventional system contribute to the relatively high running costs.

2. The inputs can be sampled at pre-selected rates which prevents the accumulation of unnecessary data. For example, it is not usually necessary to sample posture more often than once a minute. In addition there is greater control over the number and type of inputs that can be handled.

3. Rechargeable batteries can be used because the power consumption is much smaller. This also cuts running costs considerably as batteries are the single most expensive item used with the tape recorders.

4. The unit can be made more compact and lighter than the conventional one. The less obtrusive the unit, the less it will interfere with the activity of the patient.

5. Extended recording times can be used. This may allow a better overall picture of a person's activity to be obtained. In particular, there may be some advantage to having a run-in period of a few hours during which time the patient can grow accustomed to wearing the unit.

6. The unit can be directly interfaced to a microcomputer. The data can be fed directly into the computer in a matter of seconds to bypass the 24-minute playback time of tapes.

There is one major disadvantage of such a system which is that the data are processed on line and the original data are not stored; therefore the detection of artefacts is very difficult. As a result it is essential to have reliable sensors and some method for checking them. One check that can be carried out is to sample and display incoming signals at the beginning and at the end of the recording. Although this does not confirm that they have functioned correctly throughout the recording period it will help to detect some problems. There is no doubt that experience gained from the use of a tape-based system will be invaluable as an aid to understanding and avoiding problems in this area.

Fig. 8.4 shows a block diagram of a typical digital system. The heart of it is the microprocessor (MPU) which is programmed by an erasable programmable read only memory (EPROM). This can, of course, be tailored to individual requirements by reprogramming. The recorder can be programmed to sample the accelerometer channel when the person is standing up. A variable number of inputs are fed through ADCs and, after processing, the results are stored in the random access memory (RAM) which is part of the self-contained unit. When the recording is complete the unit is connected directly to the microcomputer and the results are downloaded for storage and display as before. We are currently assessing a system along these lines and although we do not expect it to be a solution to all the problems we hope that it will be an improvement on the present system. It is envisaged that such a system will have other medical applications, for example, monitoring of oesophageal pH, of patients' responses to drug therapy and of other physiological parameters.

The advantage of these ambulatory monitoring systems is that they allow patient monitoring at home where most of the problems occur. It is to be hoped that their use will allow us to gain a better understanding of patients' symptoms and diseases.

References

1 Moss NH, Dohan FC (1958) Surgical convalescence: when does it end? Ann NY Acad Sci 73: 455–464
2 Sutherland AM (1958) Psychological factors in surgical convalescence. Ann NY Acad Sci 73: 491–499
3 Rose EA, King TC (1978) Understanding post-operative fatigue. Surg Gynecol Obstet 147: 97–102
4 Editorial (1979) Post-operative fatigue. Lancet i:84
5 Christensen T, Bendix T, Kehlet H (1982) Fatigue and cardio-respiratory function following abdominal surgery. Br J Surg 69: 417–419

6 Christensen T, Kehlet H (1984) Post-operative fatigue and changes in nutritional state. Br J Surg 71: 473–476

7 Wood CD (1981) Post-operative exercise capacity following nutritional support with hypotonic glucose. Surg Gynecol Obstet 152: 39–42

8 Edwards H, Rose EA, King TC (1982) Post-operative deterioration in muscle function. Arch Surg 117: 899–901

9 Arnold DL, Bore PJ, Radda GK, Styles P, Taylor DJ (1984) Excessive intracellular acidosis of skeletal muscle on exercise in a patient with post-viral exhaustion/fatigue syndrome. Lancet *i*: 1367–1369

10 Waller AD (1885) Experiments and observations relating to the process of fatigue and recovery. Br Med J 2: 135–148

11 Waller AD (1891) The sense of effort: an objective study. Brain 14: 179–249

12 Church JM, Choong SY, Hill JL (1984) Abnormalities of muscle metabolism and histology in malnourished patients awaiting surgery: effects of a course of intravenous nutrition. Br J Surg 71: 563–569

13 Thorstensson A (1976) Muscle strength, fibre types and enzyme activities in man. Acta Physiol Scand [Suppl] 443: 7–45

14 Russell D. McR, Prendergast PJ, Darby PL, Garfinkel PE, Whitwell J, Jeejeebhoy KN (1983) A comparison between muscle function and body function in anorexia nervosa: the effect of refeeding. Am J Clin Nutr 38: 229–237

15 Scott J, Huskisson EC (1976) Graphic representation of pain. Pain 2: 175–184

16 Borg G (1970) Perceived exertion as an indicator of somatic stress. Scand J Rehabil Med 2: 92–98

17 Edwards RHT, Young A, Hosking GP, Jones DA (1977) Human skeletal muscle function: description of tests and normal values. Clin Sci Mol Med 52: 283–290

18 Klidjian AM, Foster KJ, Kammerling RM, Cooper A, Karren SJ (1980) Relation of anthropomorphic and dynamometric variables to serious postoperative complications. Br Med J 281: 899–901

19 Astrand PO (1952) Experimental studies of physical working capacity in relation to sex and age. Munksgaard, Copenhagen

20 Bink B, Bonjer FH, Van Der Sluys H (1966) Assessment of the energy expenditure by indirect time and motion study. In: Gunner, Borg (Eds), Physical activity in health and disease. Scandanavian University books, Stockholm, pp 207–214

21 MacGregor J (1979) The objective measurement of physical performance with long-term ambulatory physiological surveillance equipment (LAPSE). In: Proceedings of the third international symposium on ambulatory monitoring. Academic Press, London, pp 29–38

22 Bassey EJ, Bryant JC, Fentem PH, MacDonald IA, Patrick JM (1979) Customary physical exercise in elderly men and women using long-term ambulatory monitoring of ECG and footfall. In: Proceedings of the third international symposium on ambulatory monitoring. Academic Press, London, pp 425–432

23 Dion JL, Fouillot JP, Leblanc A (1981) Ambulatory monitoring of walking using a thin capacitive force transducer. In: Proceedings of the fourth international symposium on ambulatory monitoring. Academic Press, London, pp 420–424

24 Saltin B, Blomquist G, Mitchell JH, Johnson RL, Wildenthal K, Chapman CB (1968) Response to exercise after bed rest and after training. Circulation 38 [Suppl] 7: 1–78

25 Bassey EJ, Bennett T, Birmingham AT, Fentem PH, Fitton D, Goldsmith R (1973) Effects of surgical operation and bed rest on cardiovascular responses to exercise in hospital patients. Cardiovasc Res 7: 588–592

26 Snook R (1972) Medical aspects of ambulance design. Br Med J 3: 574–578

27 Rodahl K (1977) Physical work stress. In: Karl I, Anderson (Eds), Physical work and effort. Pergamon Press, Oxford, p 206

28 Fox III SM, Naughton JP, Haskell WL (1971) Physical activity and the prevention of coronary heart disease. Ann Clin Res 3: 404–432

29 Kinney JM, Long CL, Gump FE, Duke JH (1968) Tissue composition of weight loss in surgical patients: 1. Elective operation. Ann Surg 168: 459–474

9 Computerised Planning of Orthognathic Surgery

D.J. Birnie, N.W.T. Harradine and D. Barnard

Introduction

Orthognathic surgery is the surgical correction of jaw deformity. It may be carried out to prevent damage to soft tissue, to improve masticatory function [1,2], to improve facial appearance, or for a combination of these reasons.

Although treatment to prevent pathological damage or to improve function is an acceptable justification for surgery, reaction to people who seek to have the appearance of their faces changed surgically varies widely. Hill and Silver [3] observed that such a desire leading to consultation should be regarded as a symptom of neurosis. A number of studies have however shown that such people react rationally to a society which does not favour those with either major or minor facial deformity. Bull and Stevens [4] showed that fewer people donate less money to a charity collector with a small facial deformity and Rumsey et al. [5] demonstrated that people stand further away and on the non-disfigured side of a person with an abnormal facial appearance. Elliott et al. [6] suggested that a surgical reduction in facial deformity resulted in a more favourable assessment of attractiveness, happiness and intelligence but that this assessment developed with age and was rarely seen before 11 years.

The Development of Orthognathic Surgery

In the 1950s, the surgical correction of facial deformity was a relatively uncommon procedure. Surgery was directed primarily at the correction of dental occlusion and therefore often referred to as orthodontic surgery. The change in facial form was incidental and often not to the benefit of the patient. Such surgical treatment was regarded as an alternative to orthodontic treatment particularly in the adult patient and combined orthodontic and surgical treatment was rare. Surgery often involved the movement of dento-alveolar segments without fundamentally changing the skeletal base. The Wassmund procedure [7] for the correction of Class 2 division i malocclusion was carried out by posterior movement of the upper labial segment following the removal of the upper first premolars and a transverse ostectomy; this eliminated abnormally large overjets but in cases of mandibular hypoplasia resulted in a disastrous facial profile referred to as the Wassmund lip. Surgical correction of skeletal discrepancy of the jaws was restricted to setting back the mandible by body ostectomy, a procedure which often produced a poor occlusal result, was limited in providing correction of the skeletal anomaly and was accompanied by significant postoperative morbidity.

The introduction of the bilateral sagittal osteotomy by Obwegeser [8] and modified by Dal Pont [9] was a significant improvement on the body ostectomy and enabled anterior and posterior movement and rotation of the mandibular basal bone. The technique encouraged bony healing, offered improved stability following surgery and, most importantly, allowed forward movement of the mandible without the need for bone grafting. This made mandibular advancement a more practical procedure and allowed a good facial profile to be obtained.

Correction of skeletal open bite remained a problem. Although the sagittal split osteotomy could be used to correct a skeletal open bite with an upward rotation of the mandibular base, the long-term results were disappointing due to relapse. Limited open bites could be corrected with the Kole anterior segmental osteotomy [10] to set up the lower labial segment or the Schuchardt procedure [11] to intrude the maxillary buccal segments, but these had limited application and success in treating a skeletal anomaly which frequently lay in the maxilla [12].

Skeletal base surgery was restricted to the mandible because the alternative of total maxillary ostectomy at the Le Fort 1 level was a technically difficult procedure. Concern about the maintenance of the blood supply to the osteotomised segment dictated that the bony surgery was carried out through vertical incisions and subperiosteal bony tunnelling. The restricted access of this approach limited vertical movement of the upper jaw as osteotomy was possible but ostectomy was not. Bell [13] demonstrated through animal studies that the blood supply to the Le Fort 1 segment was maintained even where a vestibular soft tissue incision was made from first molar to first molar. After the osteotomy was completed the whole Le Fort 1 segment could be down fractured thus allowing superior and inferior (with bone grafting) repositioning of the tooth-bearing segment to correct vertical facial dysplasias [14].

Planning Orthognathic Surgery

The development of many different surgical techniques to correct facial deformity emphasised the need for careful presurgical planning if optimum facial and occlusal results were to be obtained. Although originally only study models had been used to plan surgery, surgical planning soon utilised both lateral skull radiographs and 1 : 1 lateral photographs. There are three traditional methods of planning which use either or both of these methods.

Sectioned Photographs. These involve sectioning 1 : 1 lateral photographs to simulate the final result. This method does not accurately simulate the differential movement of tissue within each segment and step defects are produced between the cuts. There are no hard tissue cephalometric data on the final result and soft tissue measurements are impeded by the step defects.

Freehand Alteration of Tracings. Epker and Fish [12] recommended the alteration of lateral skull tracings as a means of planning orthognathic surgery. The process involves constructing two tracings together with a third tracing of those structures to be moved by surgery and is very time-consuming. It is also difficult to incorporate the best available data on soft tissue changes. The technique requires some artistic skill and lacks standardisation between operators.

Combined Tracing and Photograph. Henderson [15] described the use of a combined tracing and photographic transparency. This provides a poorer predicted soft-tissue outline than the second method but allows photographic representation of the final result.

The Development of On-Line Digitising

Cephalometric analysis is tedious when it involves a large number of points, geometrical constructions and the measurement of many linear and angular distances. It was therefore a logical application for computerisation although early digitising systems were off-line. In the late 1970s, the falling price and the increased power of desk-top computers made on-line digitising practical [16]. The advantages of on-line digitising were that it allowed immediate analysis of the lateral skull radiograph and concurrent error checking. The simplest systems used very small computers with tape storage media, linked to an X–Y digitiser to measure lateral skull radiographs [17] although these were rapidly superseded by more powerful machines connected to digitisers, graphics plotters and printers. Although initially on-line digitising was restricted to simple cephalometric analysis, it was a logical step to develop programs to simulate the planning process for orthognathic surgery [18].

Hardware Requirements for On-Line Digitising and Plotting Systems

Early systems used a variety of hardware and as commercial software is not available for these applications, there was little standardisation of hardware or operating systems and much duplication of effort in writing software. Some of the hardware chosen was unsuitable for use in such systems.

The choice of hardware depends on its ability to perform the desired task, its availability for purchase, the availability of servicing and its perceived value for money. In particular the choice of digitiser is important in relation to digitising lateral skull radiographs; the digitiser must be translucent without overtly displaying any electromagnetic grid wires in the digitising table, and have an absolute accuracy of better than 0.15 mm [16]. Similarly, in choosing a graphics plotter it is desirable to have a similar resolution, a pen speed of approximately 40 cm/second and the facility to select under software control one of six or more pens.

Development of a Computerised Planning System

The system was developed in 1982 from a series of programs written for postgraduate orthodontic students at the Eastman Dental Hospital who were studying for their Master of Science degree at the University of London. Individualised cephalometric analysis programs were written for each student based on a master program. The master program was developed and extended to include planning modules. The program was originally developed on a Hewlett-Packard HP-85 microcomputer which had only 32 K of RAM and thus it was necessary to write a suite of programs which chained into each other.

The hardware currently used is as follows:

A Hewlett-Packard HP-86B microcomputer with 256 K RAM, 3.5″ flexible disc drives and a 10 Mb Winchester disc. The operating system of the HP 86B is enhanced with a plotter ROM, a matrix ROM, an advanced programming ROM and an I/O ROM.

A GTCO Digipad 5 11″×11″ translucent digitising table

A Hewlett Packard 7475A six-pen A3/A4 plotter

An Epson FX-80 dot matrix printer

The peripherals are linked together through an HPIB interface (IEEE 488–1978) as shown in Figs 9.1 and 9.2

The programs were written in the version of BASIC used in Hewlett-Packard's 80 series computers. This is an enhanced BASIC which allows the use of subprograms and matrix operations which are particularly helpful in mathematically intensive programs.

The program suite was designed to simulate the method of surgical planning described by Epker and Fish [12]; decisions about the choice and feasibility of surgery are left to the clinician. This is in contrast to a program described by Walters and Walters [19] in which the surgical movements necessary to produce an ideal result are selected automatically by the computer. The latter approach is based on the questionable premise that all the data required to predict the results of orthognathic surgery are obtainable from a cephalometric radiograph. The quality of information about soft tissues on the cephalometric radiograph is often poor and is better obtained from clinical examination. Additionally, in the program described by Walters and Walters the computer may suggest surgical movements which are unrealistic either because of the number of operations proposed or because the magnitude of the movements proposed is too small. This type of program is unacceptable to many clinicians because of their lack of involvement in the planning process.

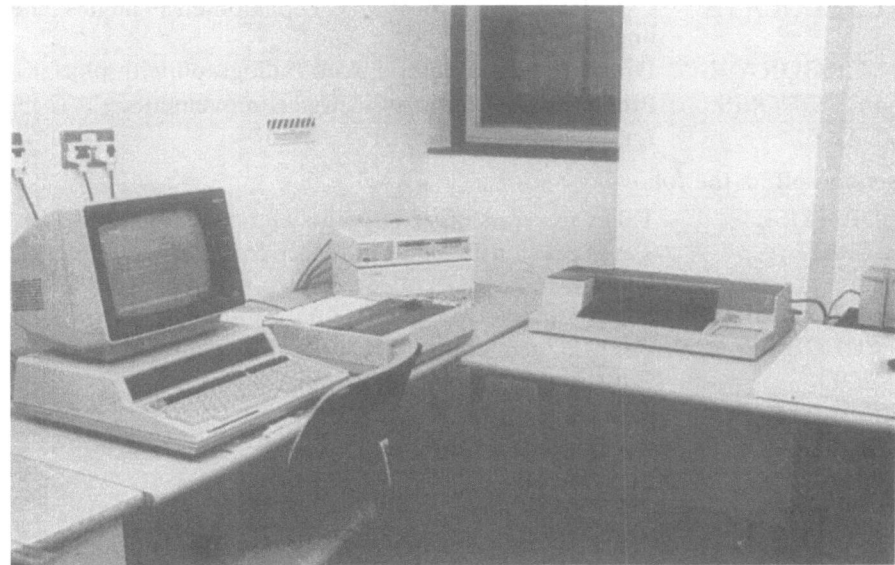

Fig. 9.1. The computerised digitising and plotting system.

Computerised Digitising and Planning System

The programs are divided into the following modules:

START   Initialise program; menu for other modules
SURGDIG   Data input and digitising

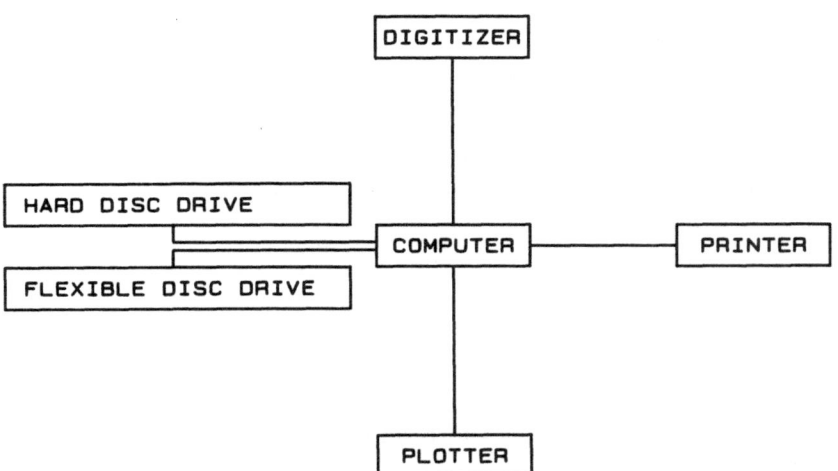

Fig. 9.2. A diagrammatic representation of the computerised digitising and plotting system.

CALCULATE   Calculates point locations, cephalometric angles and linear distances
SURGDRAW   Draws tracing of lateral skull radiograph with plotter
PROGNOSIS   Predicts orthodontic and surgical movements
LABEL   Labels plot

The menu offers the following options:

DIGITISE   Takes in cephalometric points and outlines
READ   Takes previously digitised record from disc into internal memory
SUPERIMPOSE   Superimposes two records on each other
PREDICT   Predicts orthodontic and surgical movements
EDIT   Edits a previously digitised record
DELETE   Deletes record
COPY   Backs up data onto floppy disc
LIST   Lists records

Data Entry

This is done through the digitising module. The digitising module starts by asking for the name, sex and date of birth of the patient. This is followed by the date of the X-ray to be digitised treatment and the stage to which it was taken. Treatment stages are designated as shown in Table 9.1

Table 9.1. Treatment stages in orthognathic surgery

Number	Stage
1	Start of treatment
2	Presurgical orthodontic treatment progress film
3	Immediately pre-surgery
4	End of postsurgical orthodontics
5	Retention
6	Retention

The digitiser is switched into point mode by the software for the digitisation of anatomical landmarks. The following landmarks are digitised:

Sella
Nasion
Orbitale
Porion
Condylion
Articulare
Intersection of anterior border of condylar head with base of skull
Upper incisor apex
Upper incisor tip

Lower incisor apex
Lower incisor tip
Mesial cusp of upper first molar
Distal cusp of upper first molar
Mesial cusp of lower first molar
Distal cusp of lower molar
Lower premolar point
(Upper premolar point)
Soft tissue nasion
Subnasale
Superior labial sulcus
Labrale superioris
Labrale inferioris
Lower labial sulcus

The upper premolar point is only asked for if the patient has an anterior open bite and hence upper and lower functional occlusal planes. The intersection of the anterior border of the head of the condyle is used in conjunction with articulare and condylion to determine the autorotation point of the mandible.

Once all points have been digitised, the program asks for them to be re-entered and the point locations for the first and second passes are compared. If the first and second attempts at digitising the points are more than 0.5 mm apart then that point is rejected and must be redigitised using a further two passes. This error-checking routine is repeated until all points have been recorded within the permitted tolerance. If only a single point has to be repeated then a dummy point must be digitised between successive attempts at redigitisation; the dummy point is any point at least 1 cm distant from the point being redigitised. The error-checking routine is used to reduce random error and to prevent blunders.

The digitiser switches into line mode to enter the outlines of the following anatomical structures:

Upper facial profile
Lower facial profile
Maxilla
Mandibular symphysis
Mandible
Cranial base
Nasal bone

The program calculates the coordinates of points on the outlines required for the cephalometric analysis. Thus for a record facing left, the program calculates the coordinates of posterior nasal spine (PNS) as the point with the largest x-coordinate on the maxillary outline. The program then looks back along the upper surface of the maxillary outline searching for an increasing value of the x-coordinate, and as soon as this is found the point immediately before it is taken to be anterior nasal spine (ANS). Down's A point can then be determined as the point with the largest *y*-coordinate on a coordinate system whose origin is ANS and whose *x*-axis is ANS-prosthion.

A complete list of points located from outlines is:

Soft tissue nasion
Soft tissue pogonion
Anterior nasal spine
Posterior nasal spine
Down's A point
Down's B point
Pogonion
Menton
Gonion

The cephalometric analysis is divided into six sections:

A summary analysis consisting of an 'Eastman' analysis
An analysis of the cranial base
An analysis of the shape and position of the maxilla
An analysis of the shape and position of the mandible
An analysis of the vertical components of the face
A soft tissue analysis

and provides the measurements listed in Table 9.2.

The shape of standard incisor and first molar teeth are stored in datafiles. The

Table 9.2.   Measurements from cephalometric analysis

Summary analysis			
NA	UI/MXP	MMP	OJ
NB	LI/MXP	SN/MXP	OB
NB	SNI	LFH	
Cranial base analysis			
S-N (mm)	SNBa	SN/FH	
Maxillary Analysis			
ANS-PNS	AUDH	PUDH	UI/SN
Mandibular analysis			
Co-Po (mm)	Co-Go (mm)	Go-Me (mm)	ArGoMe
ALDH	PLDH	SNPo	LI/APo
LI/APo (mm)	LI/NB	LI/NB (mm)	
Vertical analysis			
AFH (mm)	PFH (mm)	AUFH (mm)	PUFH (mm)
LAFH (mm)	PAFH (mm)	SN/MP	
Soft tissue analysis (relative to a perpendicular drawn through soft tissue nasion)			
Nasal tip (mm)	UL sulcus (mm)		Labrale superioris
Soft pogonion (mm)	LL sulcus (mm)		Labrale inferioris
LS-E line (mm)	LL-E line (mm)		Upper lip contour
Inter lip gap (mm)	Incisor exposure (mm)		Lower lip contour

upper and lower incisor outlines are scaled in length to correspond to the distance between the respective incisor tips and apices while molar outlines are used unscaled. Standard outlines are also stored for the orbital rim and porion.

The calculation of cephalometric angles and linear distances is done using linear algebra and has been described by Birnie [20]. The digitiser uses a system of Cartesian coordinates with an angular convention lying in the domain +180 degrees to −180 degrees instead of from 0 degrees to 360 degrees. It is assumed that the digitiser's own coordinate system lies at the bottom left-hand corner of the digitising table and that all x and y coordinates therefore lie in the first quadrant. This coordinate system is not necessarily the most convenient for computation and it is therefore useful to be able to transform the original coordinates to a new system with new axes and origin. The linear equations that accomplish this are:

$$x' = \cos T(x - X) + \sin T(y - Y)$$
$$y' = -\sin T(x - X) + \cos T(y - Y)$$

where X,Y is the new origin, T is the angle of rotation and x',y' are the new coordinates of the point whose original coordinates were x,y.

The same result can be achieved using matrix multiplication in the equation

$$R = M.C$$

where M is the matrix of the transformation, C is a two-element vector containing $(x - X)$ and $y - Y$ and R is the result array.

Angular measurements can be calculated using a combination of three simple geometrical rules:

The angle made by a straight line is 180 degrees

The sum of the interior angles of a triangle is 180 degrees

The exterior angle of a triangle is equal to the sum of the two interior and opposite angles

A method of calculating cephalometric values using vector algebra instead of linear algebra has been described by Konchak and Koehler [21].

Once all calculation is complete, the tracing is plotted and annotated. All plots are oriented with the Sella–Nasion line at 8 degrees to the horizontal plane of the paper and Sella has the same x and y coordinates for all records. Two qualities of plot are offered mediated through pen velocity for clinical quality plots (pen velocity = 40 cm/second) and photographic quality plots (pen velocity = 1 cm/second). The analysis printed can be either a summary analysis or the full cephalometric analysis. The option to store the data is given once the tracing is complete and program control is returned to the menu.

Superimposition of Records

SUPERIMPOSE superimposes two previously digitised records on a common coordinate system. These two records may either be serial cephalometric radiographs of the same patient or one of them may be a Broadbent–Bolton Standard [22] chosen either to match the patient's age (range 10 to 18 years) or the length of the Sella–Nasion line.

Superimposition of serial cephalometric radiographs of the same patient are usually carried out on the best fit of the anterior cranial bases, the maxillae or the mandibles. The superimposition is recorded using fiducial points. The process of superimposing two records using the mandibular plane as a reference line and given the two fiducial points is as follows:

1. The coordinates of the first radiograph are transformed to a coordinate system whose origin is Menton and whose x-axis is Gonion–Menton. This establishes the reference plane.

2. Calculate the coordinates of Menton and Gonion on the first radiograph for a coordinate system whose origin is the mid-point of the fiducial points and whose x-axis is the line joining them and call them Me(R) and Go(R). This establishes the relationship of the reference plane to the fiducial markers.

3. Transform the coordinates of the second radiograph to a coordinate system whose origin is the midpoint of its fiducial points and whose x-axis is the line joining them.

4. Transform the coordinates of the second radiograph to a coordinate system whose origin is Me(R) and whose x-axis is Me(R) to Go(R).

Planning and Prediction of Results of Surgery

Orthognathic surgery usually consists of a period of pre-surgical orthodontics, the osteotomy and fixation and a period of postsurgical orthodontics to detail the occlusion. The program allows planning of the pre-surgical orthodontics and osteotomies using movements listed in Table 9.3.

Table 9.3.   Presurgical orthodontics and osteotomies

Orthodontics	
Upper incisor movement	Retroclination, proclination, intrusion and extrusion
Lower incisor movement	Retroclination, proclination, intrusion and extrusion
Upper first molar movement	Horizontal movement along occlusal plane, intrusion and extrusion
Lower first molar movement	Horizontal movement along occlusal plane, intrusion and extrusion
Level lower occlusal plane	
Osteotomies	
Maxillary segmental	Mandibular segmental
Le Fort 1 osteotomy	Mandibular advancement or set-back
Reduction of augmentation genioplasty	

The algorithm for levelling the lower occlusal plane involves calculating the depth of the lower curve of Spee at the lower premolar point, extruding the lower premolar half of this distance to create the new lower occlusal plane, intruding the lower incisor to lie on the plane and rotating the lower first molar about its furcation so that its occlusal surface lies on the new occlusal plane. The mandible is then autorotated so that the molar teeth contact.

The segmental osteotomies are labial segment osteotomies and offer horizontal and vertical movement of the segment with or without rotation and may be planned alone or in conjunction with maxillary and/or mandibular movement.

Planning a Le Fort 1 osteotomy involves defining the horizontal movement of the maxilla (relative to the Frankfort plane), and its vertical movement and rotation by vertical change of ANS and PNS. These parameters may be defined by the operator or the program may simply be instructed to place the maxilla in a Class 1 relationship with the mandible.

Similarly, mandibular advancement or setback may be defined in terms of horizontal movement relative to the Frankfort horizontal plane or the program will place the osteotomised segment in a Class 1 relationship with the maxilla.

Finally the option to carry out a reduction or augmentation genioplasty is offered by sliding the chin segment parallel to the horizontal plane.

Soft Tissue Adjustment

The alteration of the soft tissues in response to either orthodontic tooth movement or surgical movement of basal bone does not follow a $1:1$ relationship. The soft tissue changes related to commonly used operations have been well-documented whereas for some other operations data are incomplete or unavailable. The factors for soft-tissue changes in this program were derived from weighted means of figures quoted by the following authors: Bell and Dann [23], Bell and Sheideman [24], Bloom [25], Busquets and Sassouni [26], Dann et al. [27], Epker [28], Harris [29], Hershey and Smith [30], Hohl and Epker [31], Kajikawa [32], Kent and Hinds [33], Lines and Stenhauser [34], McDonnell et al. [35], Robinson et al. [36], Rudee [37], Sheideman et al. [38], Suckiel and Kohn [39] and Willmot [40].

Little or no information exists about the soft tissue changes involved in multiple procedures and the effects of these were therefore considered to be cumulative.

Example

The patient shown in Figs 9.3a,b,c complained of difficulty in eating due to the protrusion of her upper front teeth. Examination showed her to have a Class 2 skeletal pattern with a severe Class 2 division i incisor relationship and vertical maxillary excess. There was excessive exposure of the upper incisors and associated gingival tissues and the lips were incompetent as a result of the horizontal and vertical skeletal anomalies. The upper arch was well aligned and intact but both lower second premolars had been extracted (Figs 9.4a,b,c). The computerised tracing and cephalometric analysis of the start of treatment lateral skull radiograph is shown in Fig. 9.5a and the computerised prediction of the combined orthodontic and surgical result based on the decompensation of the incisors, superior maxillary repositioning of 8 mm measured at the incisor tip and a mandibular advancement are shown in Fig. 9.5b.

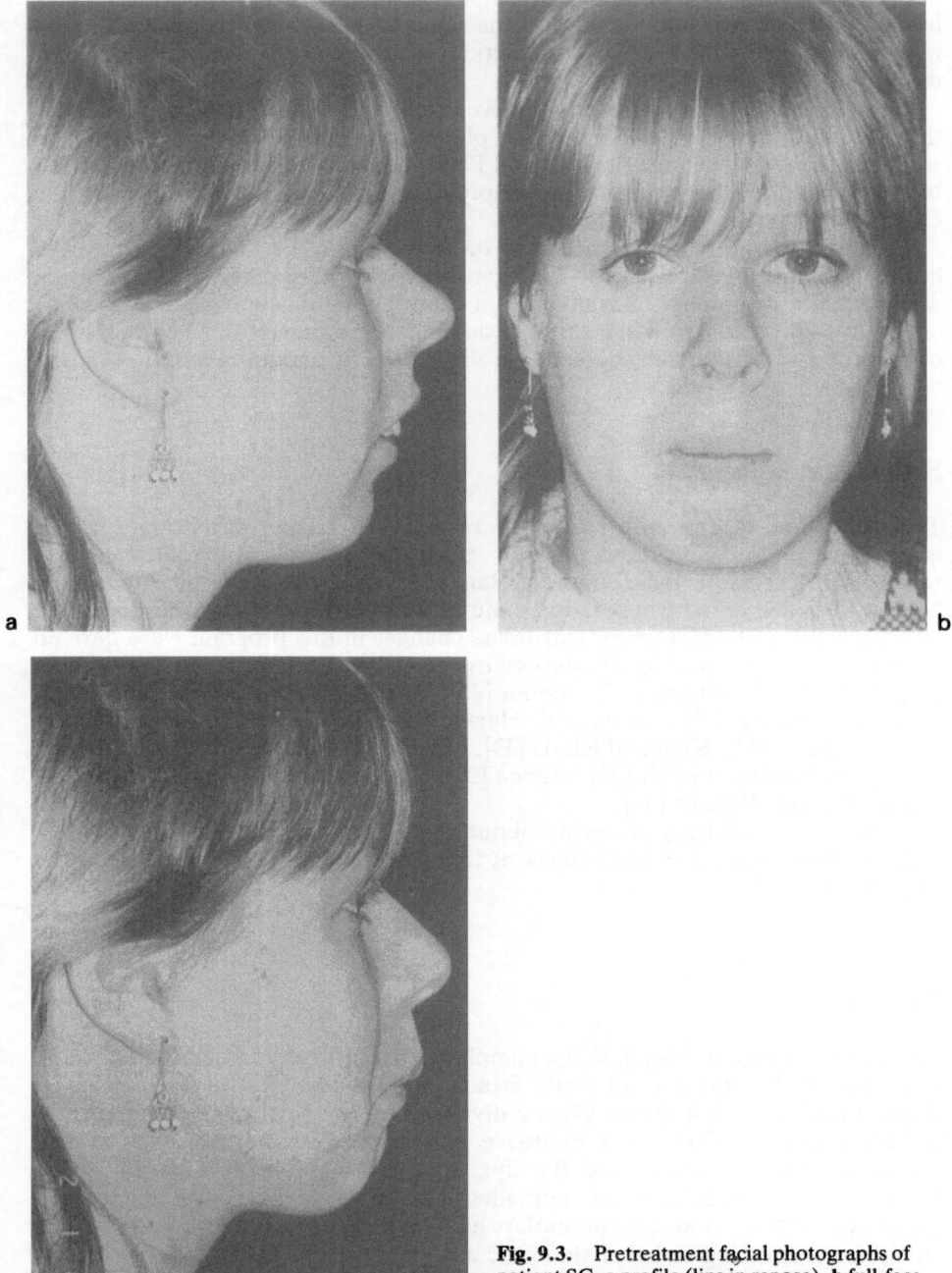

Fig. 9.3.   Pretreatment facial photographs of patient SC. **a** profile (lips in repose), **b** full-face and **c** profile (lips together).

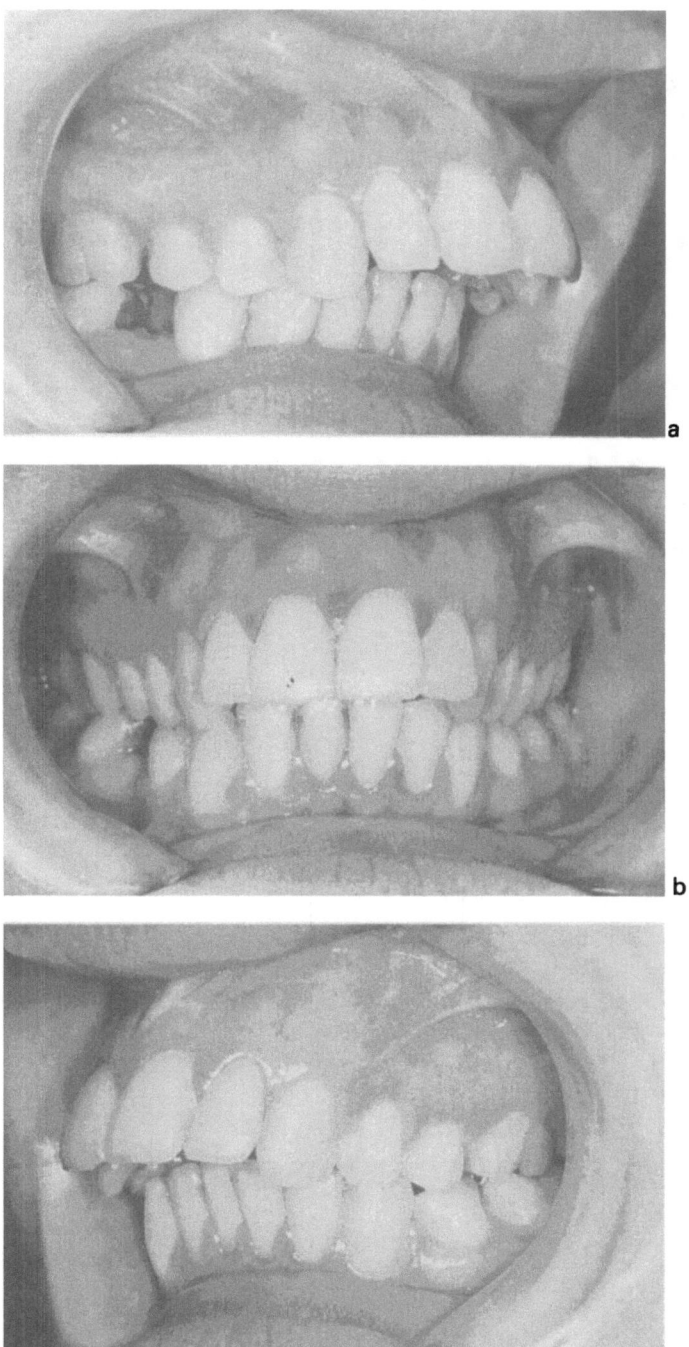

Fig. 9.4. Dental photographs of patient SC with the teeth in centric occlusion before treatment. **a** Right occlusal, **b** centre occlusal and **c** left occlusal.

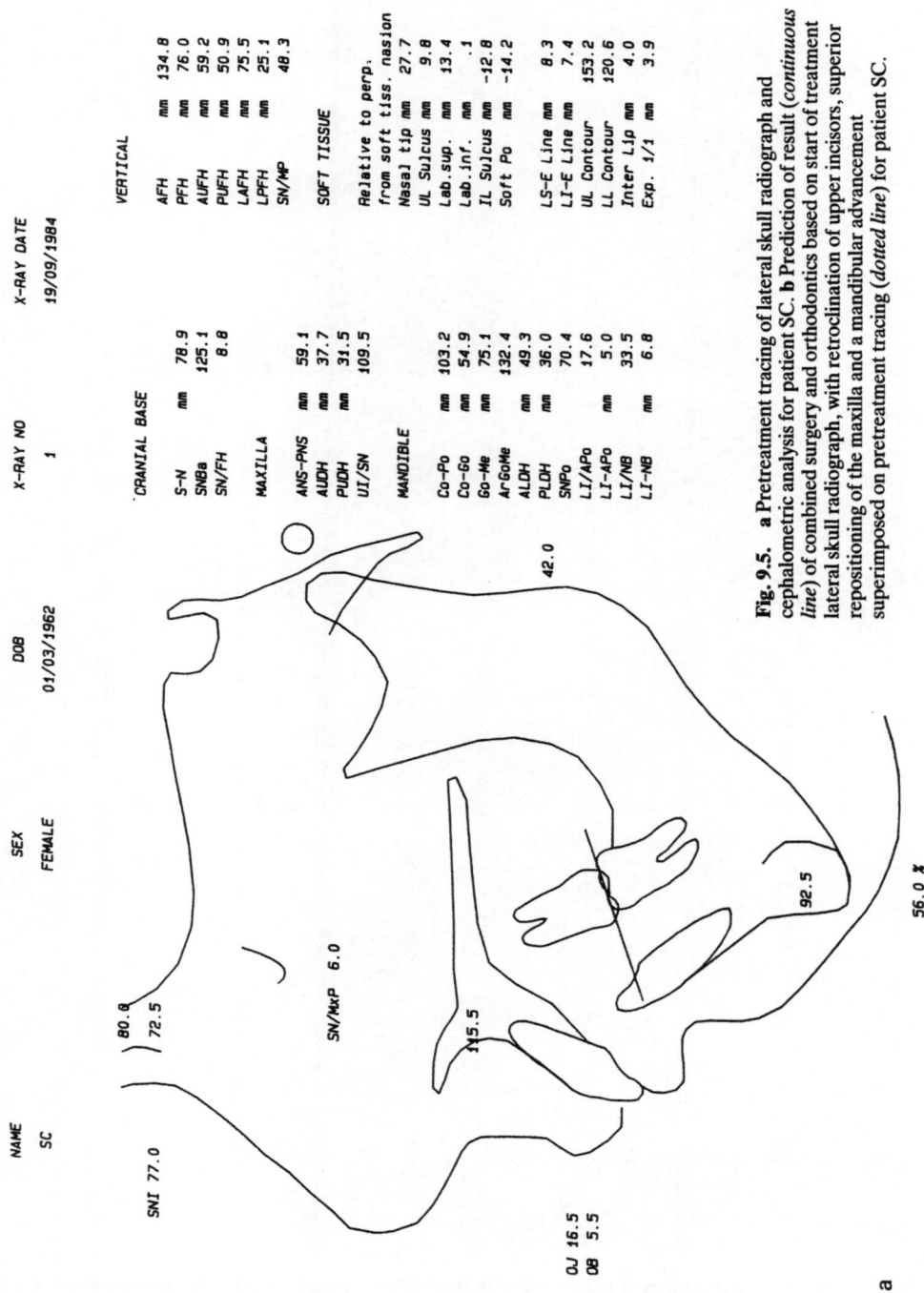

Fig. 9.5. **a** Pretreatment tracing of lateral skull radiograph and cephalometric analysis for patient SC. **b** Prediction of result (*continuous line*) of combined surgery and orthodontics based on start of treatment lateral skull radiograph, with retroclination of upper incisors, superior repositioning of the maxilla and a mandibular advancement superimposed on pretreatment tracing (*dotted line*) for patient SC.

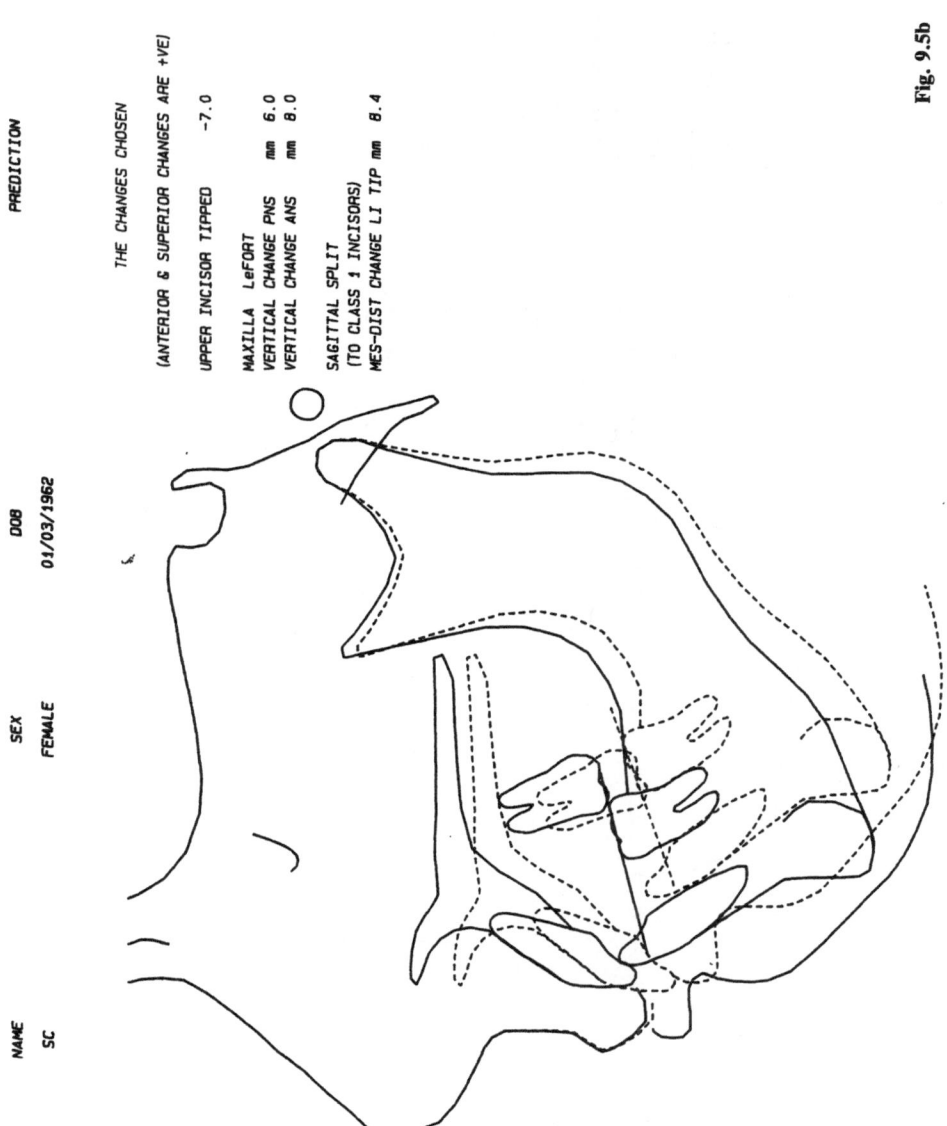

PREDICTION

THE CHANGES CHOSEN

(ANTERIOR & SUPERIOR CHANGES ARE +VE)

UPPER INCISOR TIPPED   -7.0

MAXILLA   LeFORT
VERTICAL CHANGE PNS   mm 6.0
VERTICAL CHANGE ANS   mm 8.0

SAGITTAL SPLIT
(TO CLASS 1 INCISORS)
MES-DIST CHANGE LI TIP mm 8.4

NAME
SC

SEX
FEMALE

DOB
01/03/1962

Fig. 9.5b

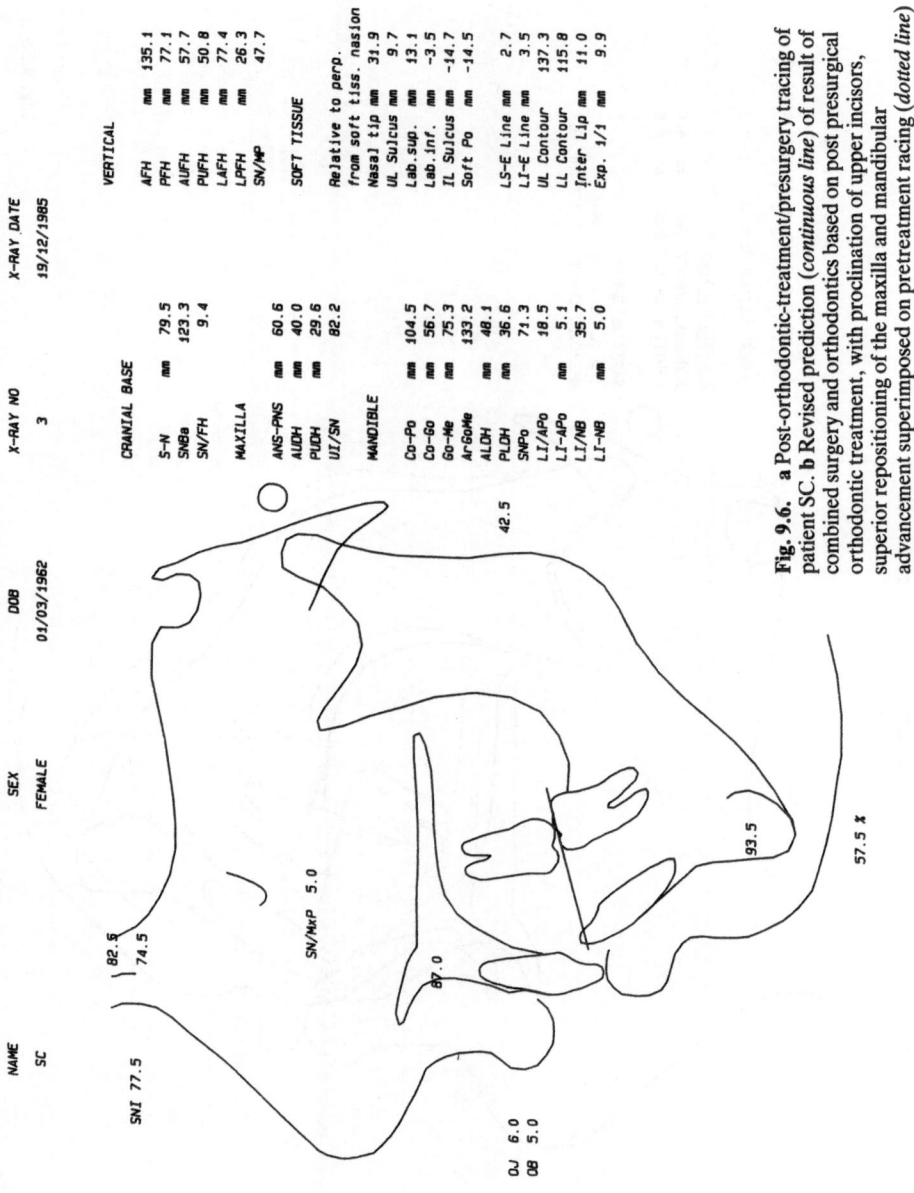

Fig. 9.6. a Post-orthodontic-treatment/presurgery tracing of patient SC. b Revised prediction (*continuous line*) of result of combined surgery and orthodontics based on post presurgical orthodontic treatment, with proclination of upper incisors, superior repositioning of the maxilla and mandibular advancement superimposed on pretreatment racing (*dotted line*) for patient SC.

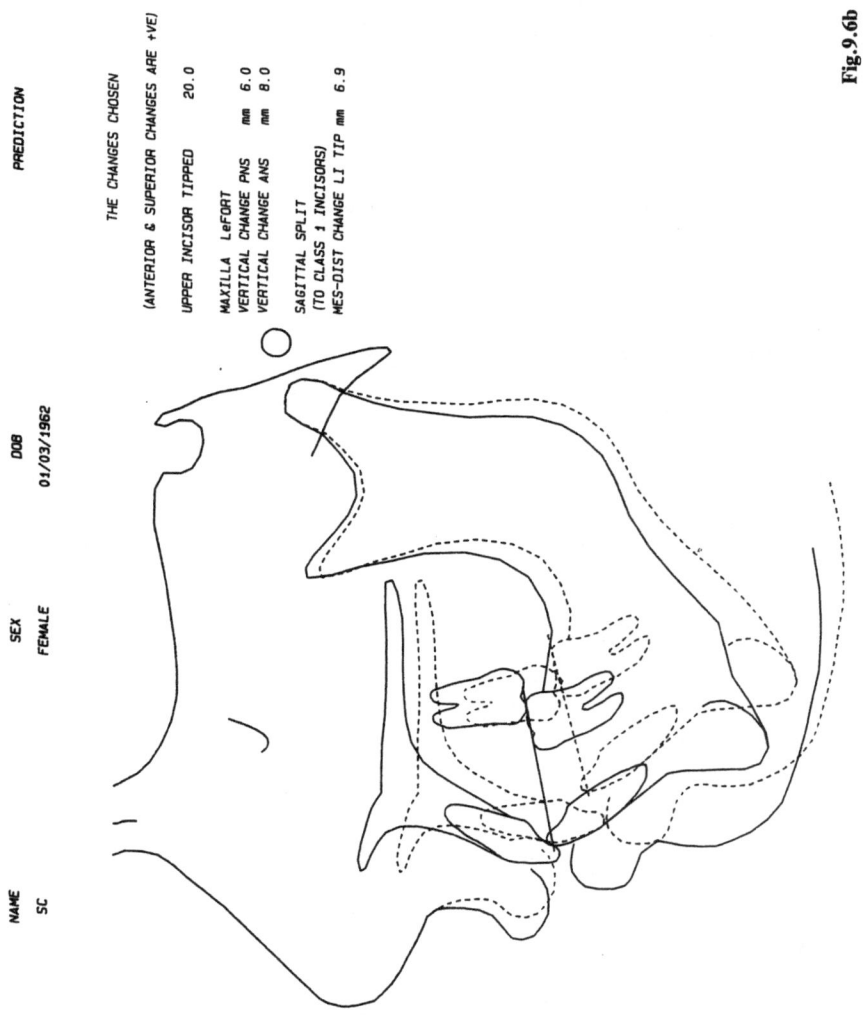

NAME
SC

SEX
FEMALE

DOB
01/03/1962

PREDICTION

THE CHANGES CHOSEN

(ANTERIOR & SUPERIOR CHANGES ARE +VE)

UPPER INCISOR TIPPED   20.0

MAXILLA LeFORT
VERTICAL CHANGE PNS   mm   6.0
VERTICAL CHANGE ANS   mm   8.0

SAGITTAL SPLIT
(TO CLASS 1 INCISORS)
MES-DIST CHANGE LI TIP mm   6.9

Fig.9.6b

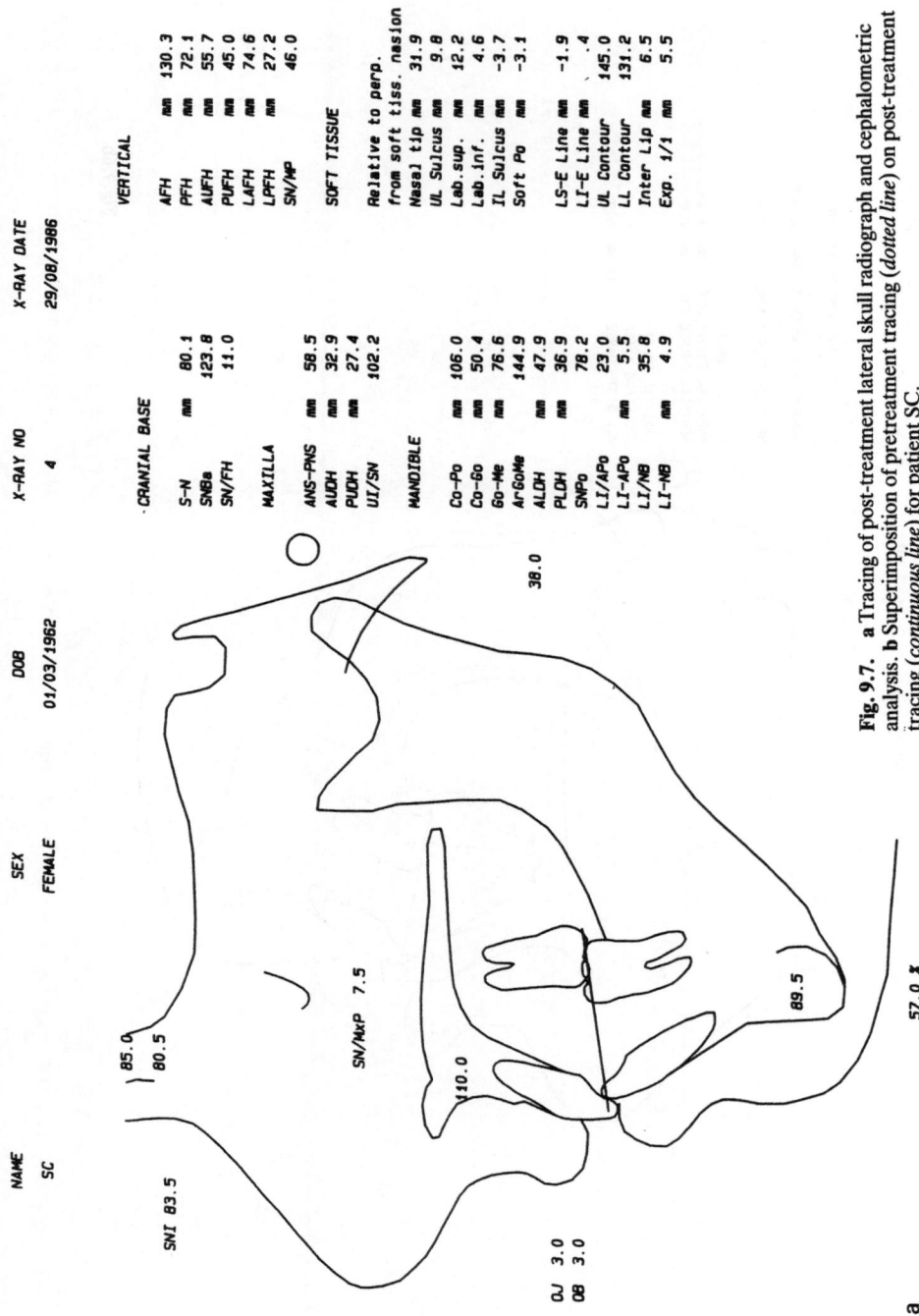

Fig. 9.7. a Tracing of post-treatment lateral skull radiograph and cephalometric analysis. **b** Superimposition of pretreatment tracing (*dotted line*) on post-treatment tracing (*continuous line*) for patient SC.

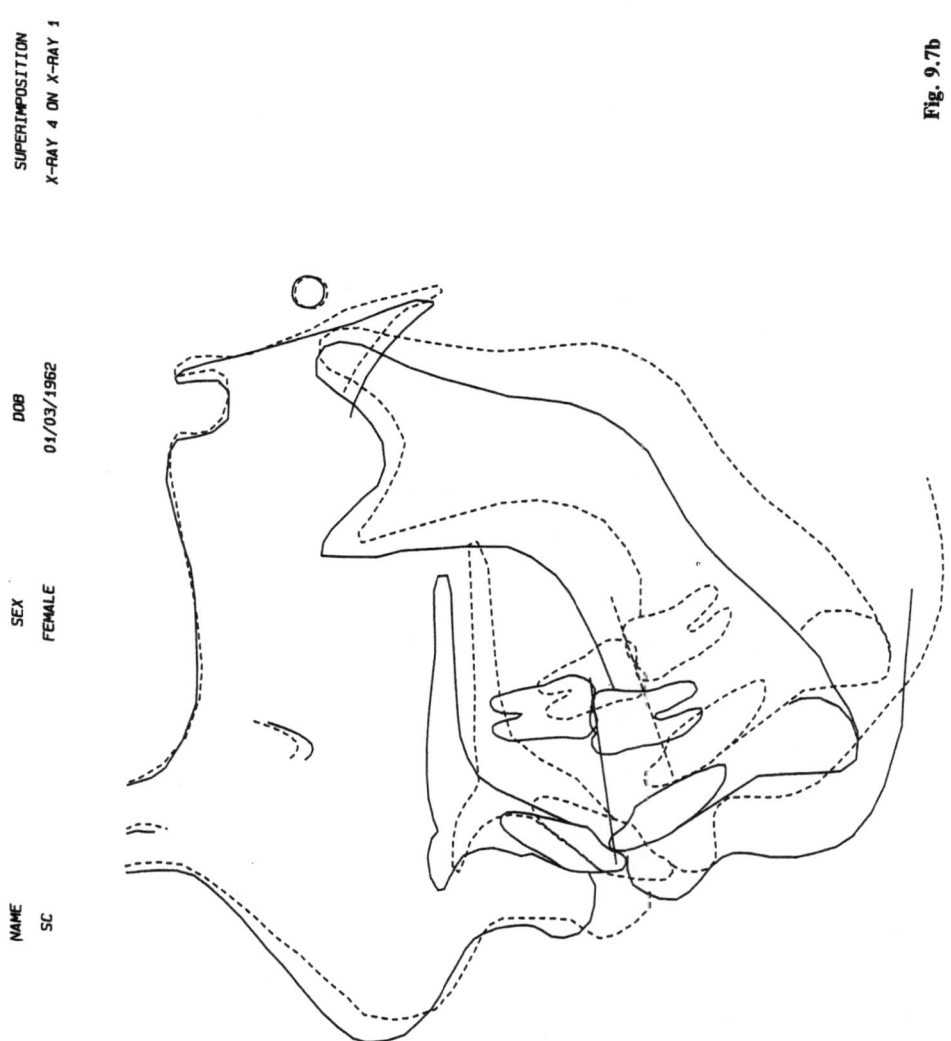

SUPERIMPOSITION
X-RAY 4 ON X-RAY 1

DOB
01/03/1962

SEX
FEMALE

NAME
SC

Fig. 9.7b

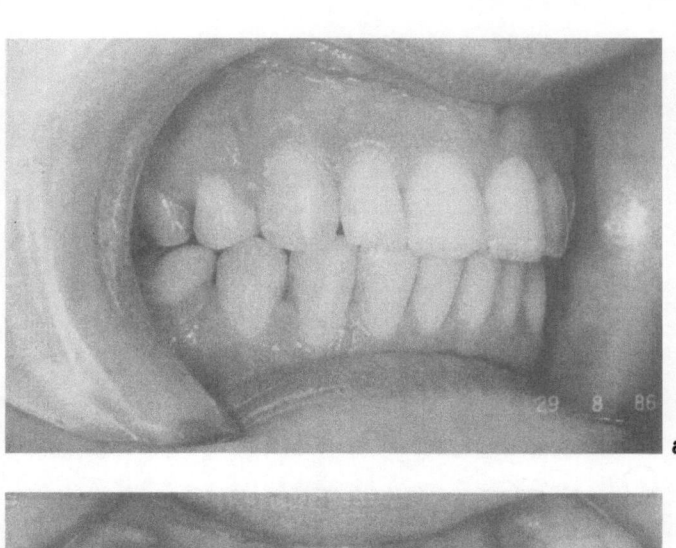

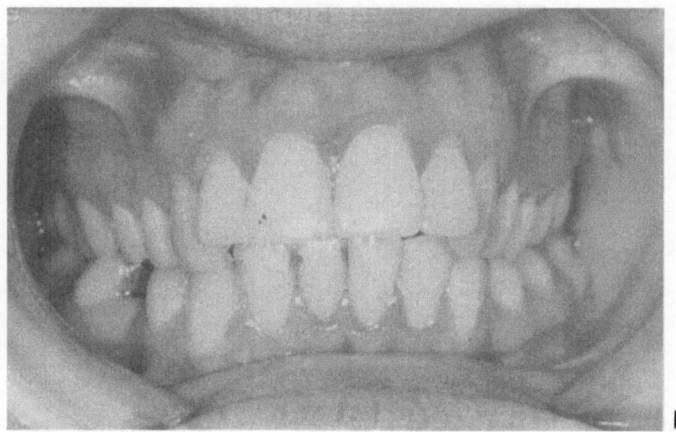

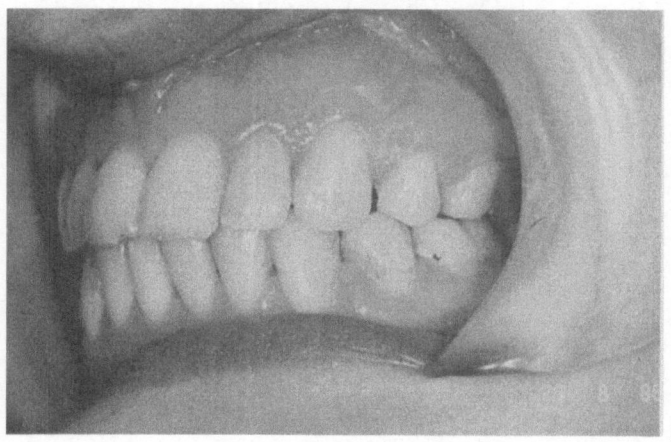

Fig. 9.8a–c. Post-treatment photographs with teeth in centric relation for patient SC. **a** Right occlusal, **b** centre occlusal and **c** left occlusal.

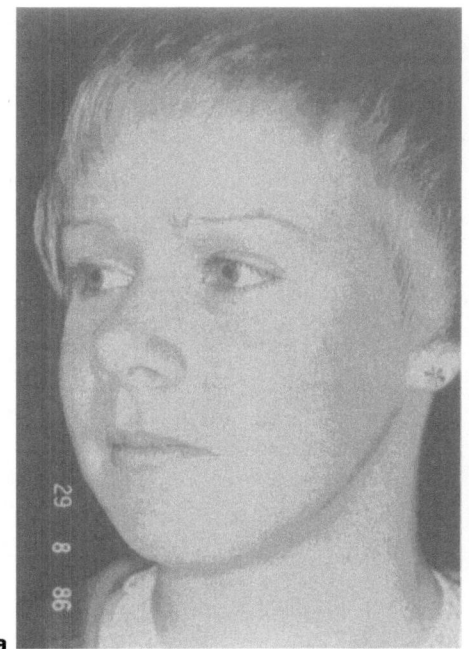

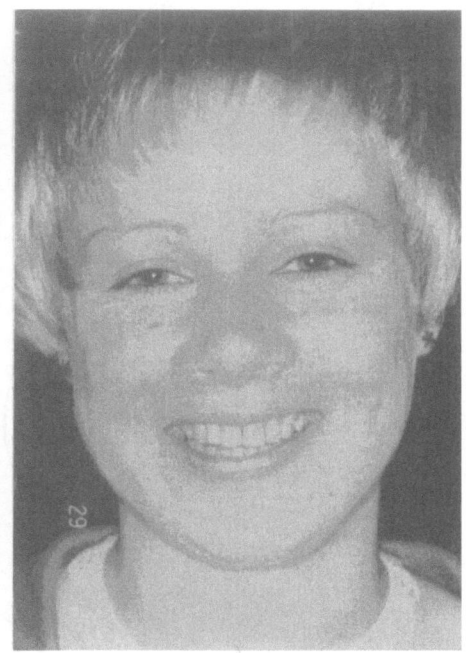

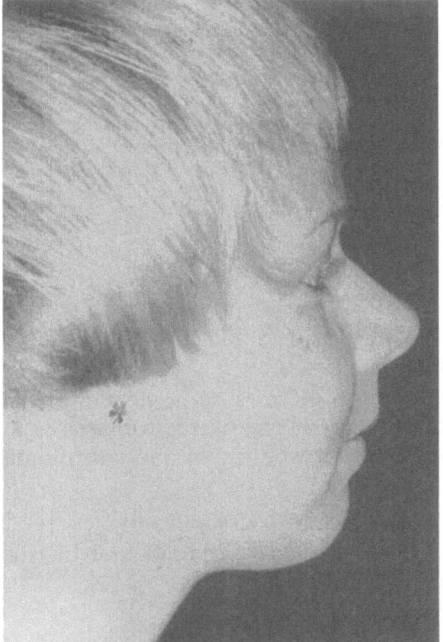

Fig. 9.9a–c. Post-treatment facial photographs of patient SC. **a** Three-quarter profile, **b** full-face and **c** profile.

| NAME | SEX | DOB | SUPERIMPOSITION |
| SC | FEMALE | 01/03/1962 | X-RAY 4 ON X-RAY P |

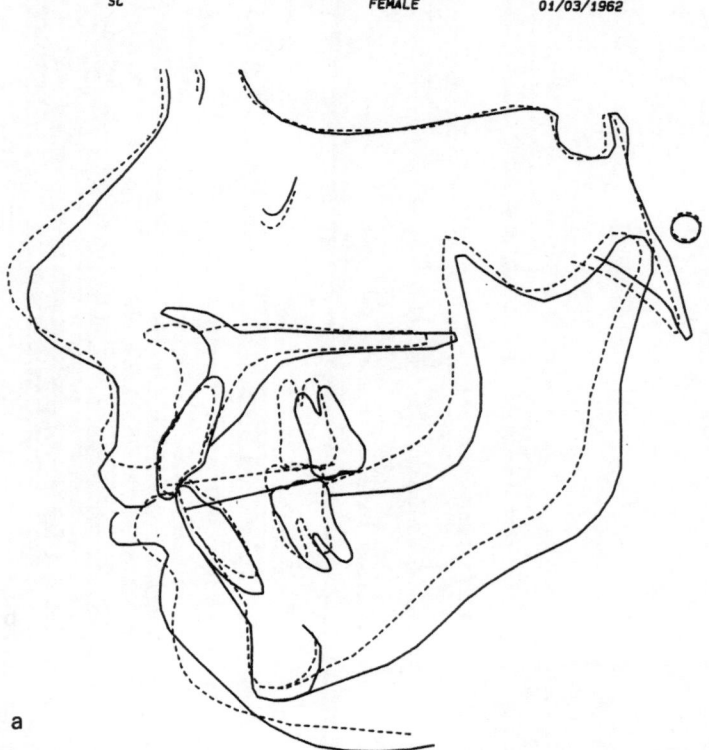

a

Fig. 9.10. a Pretreatment prediction (*continuous line*) superimposed on post-treatment tracing (*dotted line*) for patient SC. **b** Post-orthodontic-treatment/presurgery prediction (*continuous line*) superimposed on post-treatment tracing (*dotted line*) for patient SC. **c** First prediction (*dotted line*) superimposed on second prediction (*continuous line*).

The treatment plan was as follows:

1. Extraction of both upper first premolars
2. Presurgical orthodontics to retract the upper incisors to a normal axial inclination, decompensate the lower incisors, close the extraction spaces in the upper and lower arches, level the upper and lower arches and coordinate the arch form of the upper and lower arches
3. Superior repositioning of the maxilla using a Le Fort 1 osteotomy
4. Mandibular advancement to produce a normal buccal segment and incisor relationship
5. Postsurgical orthodontics to detail the occlusion
6. Retention.

The presurgical orthodontics as carried out using an 0.022″ straight-wire appliance and took approximately 12 months. Despite the use of Class 3

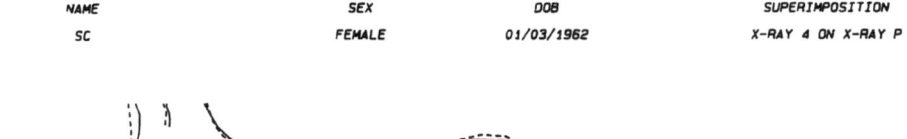

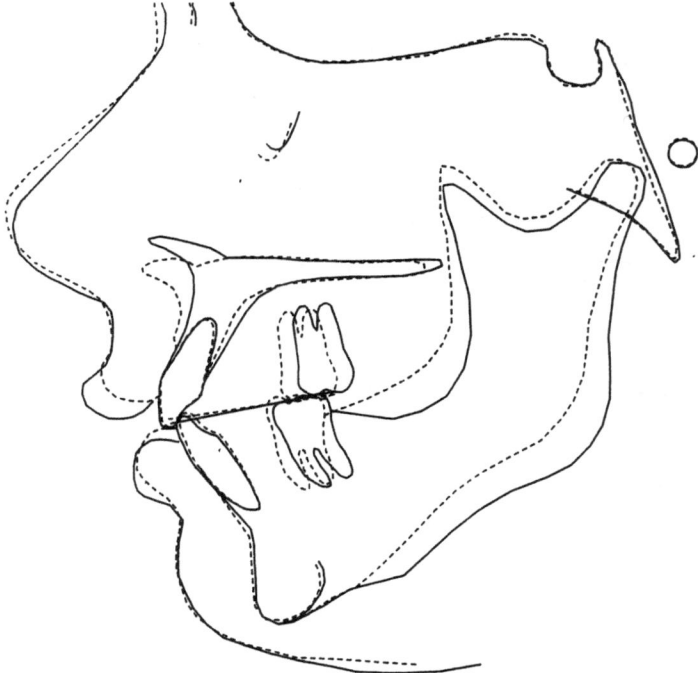

Fig. 9.10b

traction, retroclination of the upper incisors occurred which was corrected by introducing additional torque into the labial segment of an $0.019'' \times 0.025''$ stainless-steel archwire. The tracing of the lateral skull film taken two months before surgery and the revised prediction are shown in Figs 9.6a,b.

The osteotomies were carried out as planned and fixation using a carbon-fibre-reinforced acrylic intermaxillary wafer with fixation to the upper and lower fixed orthodontic appliances was continued for 8 weeks.

Postsurgical orthodontics involved the use of box elastics to close down lateral open bites and class 2 elastics to settle in the occlusion. The fixed appliances were removed 4 months after the release of the intermaxillary fixation. The final cephalometric result and the superimposition of the start and finish tracings are shown in Figs 9.7a,b, the final occlusal result in Figs 9.8a,b,c and the final facial result in Figs. 9.9a,b,c.

In Fig. 9.10a, the initial computer prediction has been superimposed on the final result and it can be seen that while the hard-tissue prediction is good, the

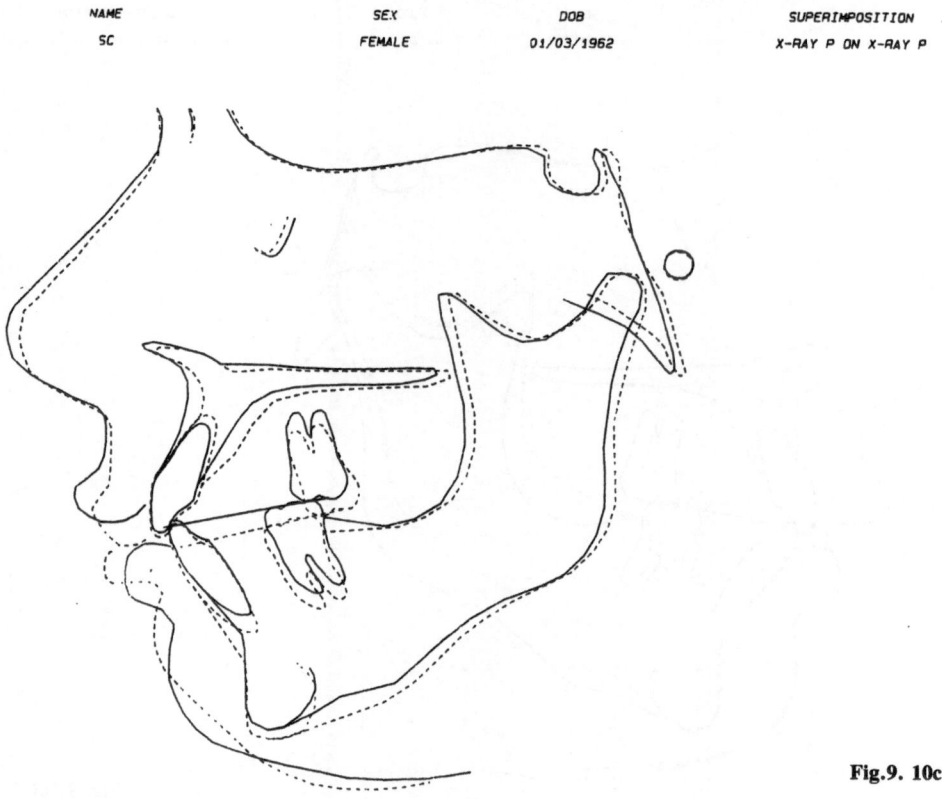

Fig. 9. 10c

soft-tissue prediction is less so. In Fig. 9.10b, the prediction performed immediately before surgery has been superimposed on the final tracing; the hard-tissue prediction remains good and the prediction of the soft-tissue profile is improved over the first attempt. This is because the latter cephalometric film was taken with the lips at rest giving the computer program better data about the shape of the lower lip to work with. In Fig. 9.10c, the first prediction has been superimposed on the second prediction.

It is not possible always to obtain optimum data about the shape and relationship of hard and soft tissue from a single cephalometric lateral skull radiograph as the relationship of the upper and lower jaws in either the retruded axis position (RAP) or the intercuspal position (ICP) may distort the shape of the upper and lower lips from their at-rest morphology.

Current Development

In 1986 the Consultant Orthodontists Group in the United Kingdom set up a working party to coordinate the development of software for orthodontics and make specific recommendations for both software and hardware. The working party has recommended the following hardware:

IBM AT microcomputer

IBM Proprinter dot matrix printer

GTCO Digipad 5 $11'' \times 11''$ translucent digitising tablet

Hewlett Packard 7440A 8 pen plotter

Software is currently available to perform basic digitising functions such as the Eastman cephalometric analysis referred to earlier and a Ricketts cephalometric analysis. The orthognathic program described above is being updated and rewritten in "C" to run on the new system.

Future Development

The present rate of hardware and software development suggests that it will soon be possible to process digital images on powerful microcomputers thus allowing direct digitising from a high resolution monitor making the X-Y digitiser unnecessary. A preliminary report on the application of digital image processing to cephalometric radiography has been published by Jackson et al. [41].

References

1 Astrand P (1974) Chewing efficiency before and after surgical correction of developmental deformities of the jaw. Swed Dent J 67: 135–145
2 Luke DA, Lucas PW (1985) Chewing efficiency in relation to occlusal and other variations in the natural human dentition. Br Dent J 159: 401–403
3 Hill and Silver (1951) Psychodynamic and aesthetic motivations for plastic surgery. Psychosom Med 12: 345
4 Bull R, Stevens J (1981) The effects of facial deformity on helping behaviour. Ital J Psychol 8: 25
5 Rumsey, N, Bull R, Gahagan D (1982) The effect of facial disfigurement on the proxemic behaviour of the general public. J Appl Soc Psychol 12: 137
6 Elliott M, Bull R, James D, Lansdown R (1986) Childrens' and adults' reactions to photographs taken before and after facial surgery. J Maxillofac Surg 14: 18–21
7 Wassmund M (1935) Lehrbuch der praktischen Surgerie des Mundes und der Kieser. Meuser, Leipzig
8 Obwegeser H, Trauner R (1957) Surgical correction of mandibular prognathism and retrognathia with consideration of genioplasty. Oral Surg 10: 677
9 Dal Pont G (1961) Retromolar osteotomy for the correction of prognathism, J Oral Surg 19: 42
10 Kole K (1959) Surgical operations on the alveolar ridge to correct occlusal abnormalities. Oral Surg 12: 277
11 Schuchardt K (1959) Experience with the surgical treatment of deformities of the jaws: prognathia, micrognathia and open bite. In: Wallace AB (ed) International society of plastic surgeons, second congress. E & S Livingstone, London
12 Epker BN and Fish LC (1978) Surgical orthodontic correction of open bite deformity. Am J Orthod 73:601–618
13 Bell WH (1973) Biological basis for maxillary osteotomies. Am J Phys Anthropol 38: 279–289
14 Bell WH, Creekmore TD and Alexander RG (1977) Surgical correction of the long face syndrome. Am Orthod J 71: 40–67
15 Henderson D (1974) The assessment and management of bony deformities of the middle and lower face. Br J Plast Surg 27: 287–296

16 Houston WJB (1979) The application of computer aided digital analysis to orthodontic records.
    Eur J Orthod 1: 71–79
17 Birnie DJ (1980) On-line digitizing: a basic system. Br J Orthod 7: 81–87
18 Harradine NWT, Birnie DJ (1986) Computerised prediction of the results of orthognathic
    surgery. J Maxillofac Surg 13: 245–249
19 Walters H, Walters DH (1986) Computerised planning of maxillo-facial osteotomies: the
    program and its clinical applications. Br J Oral Maxillofac Surg 24: 178–189
20 Birnie DJ (1983) On-line digitising: useful mathematical techniques. Br J Orthod 10: 78–89
21 Konchak PA, Koehler JA (1985) A Pascal program for digitizing lateral cephalometric
    radiographs. Am J Orthod 87: 197–200
22 Broadbent BH Senior, Broadbent BH Junior, Golden WH (1975) Bolton standards of dento-
    facial development and growth. CV Mosby, St Louis
23 Bell WH, Dann JJ (1973) Correction of dentofacial deformities by surgery in the anterior part of
    the jaws. Am J Orthod 64: 162–187
24 Bell WH, Sheideman GB (1981) Correction of vertical maxillary deficiency: stability and soft
    tissue changes. J Oral Surg 39: 666–670
25 Bloom LA (1961) Perioral profile changes in orthdontic treatment. Am J Orthod 47: 371
26 Busquets CJ, Sassouni V (1981) Changes in the integumental profile of the chin and lower lip
    after genioplasty. J Oral Surg 39: 499–504
27 Dann JJ, Fonseca RJ, Bell WH (1976) Soft tissue changes associated with total maxillary
    advancement. J Oral Surg 34: 19–23
28 Epker BN (1981) Superior repositioning of the maxilla: long term results. J Maxillofac Surg 9:237
29 Harris MC (1972) Soft tissue effects of surgical anterior maxillary retraction. Thesis for
    Certificate in Orthodontics, University of Kentucky — quoted in Bell Profitt (1980): Surgical
    correction of dentofacial deformities. Saunders, Philadelphia
30 Hershey HG, Smith LH (1974) Soft tissue profile changes associated with surgical correction of
    the prognatic mandible. Am J Orthod 65: 483–502
31 Hohl TS, Epker BN (1976) Macrogenia: a study of treatment results, with treatment
    recommendations. J Oral Surg 41: 545–567
32 Kajikawa Y (1979) Changes in soft tissue profile after correction of Class 3 malocclusion. Am J
    Orthod 37: 167–174
33 Kent JN, Hinds EC (1971) Management of dentofacial deformity by anterior alveolar surgery. J
    Oral Surg 29: 13
34 Lines PA, Steinhauser EW (1974) Soft tissue changes in relationship to movement of hard
    structures in orthognathic surgery: a preliminary report. J Oral Surg 32: 891
35 McDonnell JP, McNeill RW, West RA (1977) Advancement genioplasty: a retrospective
    cephalometric analysis of osseous and soft tissue changes. J Oral Surg 35: 640–647
36 Robinson WW, Speidel TM, Isaccson KJ, Worms FW (1972) Soft tissue profile changes produced
    by reduction of mandibular prognathism. Angle Orthod 42: 227
37 Rudee DA (1964) Proportional profile changes concurrent with orthodontic therapy. Am J
    Orthod 50: 571
38 Sheideman GB, Legan WH, Bell WH (1981) Soft tissue changes with combined mandibular
    setback and advancement genioplasty. J Oral Surg 39: 505–509
39 Suckiel JM, Kohn MW (1978) Soft tissue changes related to the surgical management of
    manidbular prognathism. Am J Orthod 73: 676–680
40 Willmot DR (1981) Soft tissue profile changes following correction of Class 3 malocclusion. Br J
    Orthod 8: 175–181
41 Jackson PH, Dickson GC, Birnie DJ (1985) Digital image processing of cephalometric
    radiographs: a preliminary report. Br J Orthod 12: 122–132

10 Computerised Total Parenteral Nutrition

S. Shami

Introduction

Total parenteral nutrition (TPN) is a relatively new technique for providing all the nutritional needs of a patient in whom oral feeding is either not possible or not desirable. The conditions where TPN has gained widest acceptance include entero-cutaneous fistulae, active inflammatory bowel disease and prolonged ileus. We have also found it very useful in the management of acute pancreatitis. More controversial indications include preoperative feeding before major procedures, short-term postoperative feeding, and as a supplement to enteral nutrition. Because of its high cost, it is necessary to select patients carefully and to provide TPN in the most cost-effective manner possible.

Principles of Parenteral Nutrition

TPN is usually given through a central venous line. This is inserted in the operating theatre under sterile conditions. A direct puncture or a cutdown into the subclavian vein is performed and the skin puncture site is separated from the venous access point by tunnelling under the chest wall skin in order to reduce line sepsis rates. The tip of the catheter ideally lies in the superior vena cava.

The complications of placing a central line are well documented and include pneumothorax, damage to proximal structures and line sepsis. Peripheral vein nutrition (PVN) is gaining wider acceptance as this eliminates the complications of a central line. Our policy is to use PVN in patients whose calculated nitrogen requirement is less than 12 g/day and where it is estimated that intravenous nutritional support will be required for less than 14 days. PVN is not practical in patients whose nitrogen requirement is over 12 g/day, as the solutions given have a high sugar content in order to stay within the recommended calorie : nitrogen ratio, and are very irritant; they should only be given into a large vein with a central line.

One of the problems with nutritional support is expense. The increasing use of large volume containers, three-litre bags, which contain all the patient's requirements over a 24-hour period has increased costs. Some manufacturers will provide ready-mixed three-litre bags of low, medium and high nitrogen content for delivery to a hospital on a regular basis. This is very convenient for hospitals where the pharmacy department does not have the facility to mix solutions in a sterile laminar flow chamber, but the disadvantage is that only standard solutions can be supplied and these may not exactly match the patient's requirements. All additives that shorten the shelf-life of these ready-mixed three-litre bags are excluded from the formulation, so that such additives must be given to the patient by a separate peripheral line, further increasing cost and inconvenience. The average cost of a ready-manufactured three-litre bag is about £60, thus large costs can be incurred in a 3-month feeding program.

Close monitoring of the program is required both for cost effectiveness and to ensure that the patient is benefitting from the TPN. The calculations needed for this are not complex but are time-consuming when done by hand or even with a calculator. Each day the following 24-hour requirements of fluid, electrolytes, nitrogen, calories and vitamins need to be determined.

Each of the fluid outputs of the patient (urine, vomit, fistula output, etc) must be collected over each 24-hour period in order to determine the nitrogen, fluid and electrolyte losses. These results are then coordinated with the input values over the same period so that the balance of each can be calculated.

A close check is maintained on the patient's general condition by repeated blood tests. The serum levels of sodium and potassium act as indicators of the intra and extra-cellular ionic balance, the serum urea levels provide an indicator of renal function and protein metabolism while routine haematology can predict the development of anaemia and incipient sepsis.

Table 10.1.   Tests needed to monitor a patient on TPN

Daily tests
   Fluid, electrolyte, nitrogen input and output
   FBC, urea and electrolytes and serum glucose
   Urinary sodium, potassium, urea and protein
   Body weight and temperature

Twice-weekly tests
   Liver function tests, calcium, phosphate and serum proteins
   Blood clotting studies
   Platelet count

Fortnightly tests
   Cholesterol and triglycerides
   Iron and TIBC
   Magnesium and zinc
   Vitamin B_{12} and folate

Table 10.1 lists all the tests that are needed to monitor a patient on TPN. If the patient's condition is unstable, or there is evidence that it is deteriorating then some of the tests may need to be done more frequently than indicated.

Computerisation of Total Parenteral Nutrition

TPN lends itself very well for computerisation because:

1. All the calculations can be done rapidly without error
2. Prescriptions for the pharmacy department listing the patient's daily requirement can be automatically generated
3. The results of blood test as well as the calculated outputs and balances can be graphically displayed so that the clinician can check on the progress of the patient
4. Request forms for blood tests and fluid-output analysis can be automatically generated
5. A computer program could act as an "Expert" on TPN in a hospital where the staff is unfamiliar with the intricacies of parenteral feeding.

Review of Current Software for TPN

Hitherto most computer programs for TPN have concentrated only on calculating the nutritional requirements of the patient, and producing a daily prescription of required solutions. These programs have mainly been written for hand-held computers for use at the bed-side. James et al. [1] in 1978 described two programs for a programmable calculator, the first of which, the requirements program, uses patient data and the results of blood and fluid-excretion analyses to calculate the patient's nutritional requirements. The second program, the bottle selection program, fits an intravenous bottle regimen to the patient's calculated requirements. Goggin [2] also in 1978 described a similar program for a Hewlett Packard programmable calculator which in addition printed out the calculated requirements with infusion rates and cost of the solutions. In 1985 Goggin and Hoskins [3] described a program running on a Commodore PET microcomputer written in BASIC which calculated a patient's requirements, selected an appropriate regimen and gave advice on how to infuse it. Anthony and Cyril Wong [4] described a similar program written in BASIC and running on an Apple computer. Two further programs running on pocket computers have been described by Colley et al. [5] and Skaredoff and Consoli [6]. Several programs have also been written for TPN in neonates and children.

Hardware

Expense has previously prevented hospital departments from acquiring microcomputers, but the price of hardware has dropped so much in recent years that a microcomputer with reasonable memory and excellent graphics capability can now be bought relatively cheaply. An IBM compatible microcomputer with a full complement of memory (640 kilobytes), a floppy disc drive, a 20-megabyte hard disc drive, colour monitor and a dot matrix printer can be obtained for about £1200. A similar system without the hard disc and with only a monochrome monitor can cost as little as £600. Thus it is now practical to write large programs which take advantage of the memory and graphic capabilities of these machines.

Software

Attempts have been made to use spreadsheet and database packages for monitoring TPN, but a good knowledge of the software is required and persons unfamiliar with computers would not be able to use such packages easily. In order to monitor TPN with a user-friendly interface the only practical solution is to write a bespoke software program. To do this a programming language best suited for this type of application needs to be selected.

Computer languages can in general be subdivided into low and high-level languages. A low-level language, such as assembler language, is a symbolic representation of the binary code that can be directly read by the computer. Such programs run extremely fast. To write in assembler, the programmer needs a very good understanding of the computer and large programs are very difficult to write and to debug (correct errors). Most programmers will use only small assembly language routines within a much larger high-level language program and then only when high speed of execution is required. An example is when data acquisition from real-time monitoring is required. The high-level languages such as BASIC (Beginner's All-purpose Symbolic Instruction Code), PASCAL, FORTRAN (FORmula TRANslation) and C facilitate the writing of programs as they are much closer to natural English. However in order to run they must first be translated by an intermediate program called an interpreter or a compiler into a sequence of binary instructions which the computer can understand. An interpreter program translates the program, line by line, as it is running and so execution speed is slow. BASIC and FORTRAN are usually interpreted languages. BASIC compilers however are now becoming available and their use can increase program execution speed by up to ten times. A compiler takes the complete program, translates it into machine code, and thus produces a completely different version of the program consisting of a series of binary instructions. This only needs to be done once and thereafter the program runs at machine-code speed each time. PASCAL and C are usually compiled languages. The disadvantage of using a compiled programming language is that each time a small part of the program is written, the whole program has to be recompiled to check for errors. If an error is found, it has to be corrected, recompiled and then checked for further errors. Compilation can be slow and so the process of debugging can be tedious and slow. With interpreted languages the process is much faster as the error can be corrected and the program re-run immediately.

Although the most popular programming language, BASIC has four main problems.

1. It is an interpreted language and thus programs written in BASIC run very slowly

2. There are many versions of BASIC and a program written in one dialect on a particular computer is unlikely to run on another type of computer without major modifications

3. BASIC is a sequential programming language which means that each line in a basic program is numbered and executed in order. This makes the writing and debugging of large programs difficult. If any enhancements are to be added at a later time they have to be squeezed into the program and all the following line numbers may have to be changed

4. BASIC does not normally support structured programming.

The meaning of this will be explained below.

BASIC is provided free with many computers and because writing small to medium sized programs using it is easy, it has retained its popularity.

PASCAL is probably the most popular compiled programming language. It produces fast compact programs and there is little variation between the various PASCAL compilers. A program written on one computer can be transferred reasonably easily to any other computer which supports a PASCAL compiler. PASCAL, unlike BASIC, supports structured programming; the main program is broken down into small blocks each being a mini-program complete in itself and addressing a specific, clearly defined objective, such as doing a series of mathematical calculations, requesting data input or displaying information on the screen. A number of blocks can then be grouped together to form a module, and one or more of these modules form the program. In this way large programs are broken up into smaller parts which can be easily written and debugged. It also promotes a logical and disciplined train of thought. PASCAL is also a declarative and strongly typed language: all variables that are going to be used in the program are declared in advance of the main program and the type of each variable defined. A variable such as (pat_name) as the name of the patient, must be declared in the declaration part of the program along with its type i.e. a string of characters. Similarly the variable (pat_age) for the age of the patient has to be declared, but in this case its type is declared as being an integer. PASCAL supports integers, real numbers, bytes, strings, characters, boolean and user defined types. This avoids confusion over variable names and adds to the clarity of the program.

Most versions of BASIC and PASCAL have a 64 kilobyte limit to the size of a program. If a program needs to exceed this limit then it has to be broken down to several separate programs of less than 64 kilobytes in length which can then be chained together to form the complete program. Chaining works in the following way: the link of the chain in current use takes over the full memory of the computer. In order to use the next link of the program the present one is wiped out of memory and the new link moves into its place. A small module is used as a calling program to bring each link of the chain from the disc into the computer memory in the correct sequence. It is important that the values of all variables used in the previous link be preserved for use in subsequent links. The modular approach used in PASCAL helps with this as the variables once declared are stored in a separate location in memory. Because the program we wanted to write lent itself to a modular approach and we required speed of execution we chose PASCAL as our programming language. We chose Turbo PASCAL Version 3.0 rather than any other PASCAL compiler for a number of reasons: it has a very fast compiler; it includes a comprehensive editor; on detection of an error on compilation the programmer is returned automatically to the editor at the source of the error; it offers many IBM-specific high-quality graphics routines in the Turbo Graphix Toolbox; and it is very cheap.

The only drawback to Turbo is that it is not a completely standard PASCAL. We decided to write the program for IBM and compatible microcomputers as these have become the industry standard in microcomputers; however all the non-standard Turbo routines and the IBM-specific routines have been written in a separate module so that, by re-writing this single module, the program can be made to run on any microcomputer that supports a PASCAL compiler.

Aim of the Program

The aim of the program was to produce a usable system that would:

1. Aid the selection of patients suitable for feeding parenterally
2. Give advice on the best method of feeding a particular patient
3. Determine the daily requirements of the patients and produce a prescription sheet for pharmacy, or select a regimen from a standard set
4. Suggest the tests needed each day
5. Calculate, display and print the fluid, nitrogen and electrolyte balances in table form and graphically
6. Keep a database of patients on TPN recording details of their progress, their TPN access lines, and complications, for use as an audit of the TPN services of the unit
7. Reduce the amount of time spent by the junior medical staff in the management of the patients
8. Make the management of TPN educational

TPN Timetable

Before computerising TPN we had to standardise our data collection, and so we set up a TPN Timetable (Fig. 10.1) which was circulated to junior doctors, ward sisters, pharmacy and laboratories.

At 6 a.m. the previous 24-hour collection of each of the fluids passed by the patient is completed. The volume of each output is determined and recorded and the collection of outputs for the next 24-hour period is commenced. This time was chosen because it is convenient for the nurses.

At 8 a.m. the house surgeon enters the previous day's input and output of fluid and electrolytes into the computer. The input is simply the volume of the TPN plus any other solutions that were given. From this the nitrogen and electrolyte infused are automatically calculated by the computer. The output is the volume charted by the nurses. The electrolyte content of the urine is taken as the previous day's spot urine test mentioned below. Default values are used for the estimation of the electrolyte content of the other outputs. Using this information the next day's requirement is automatically calculated. A prescription sheet is printed by the computer and sent to the pharmacy. A print-out giving a list of the

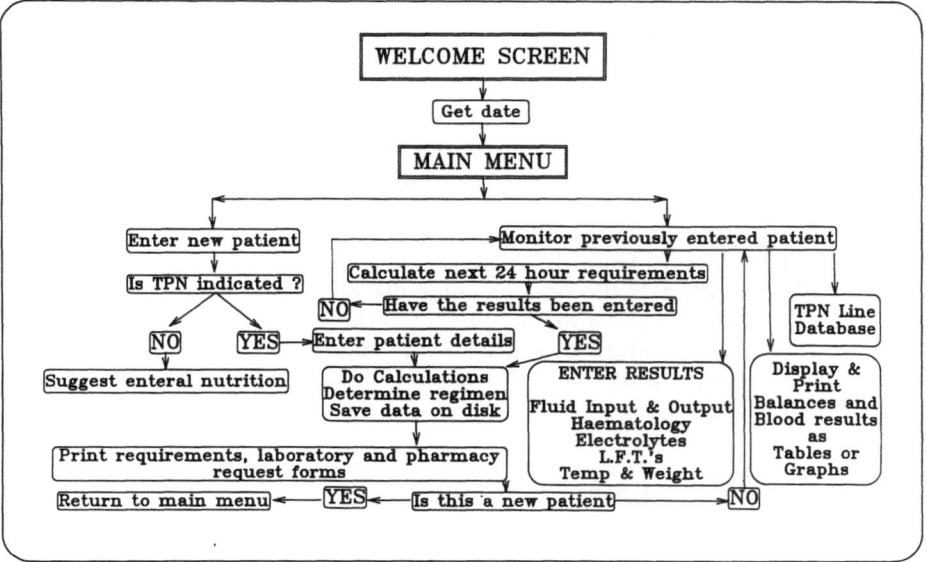

Fig. 10.1. Daily timetable for total parenteral nutrition.

blood and urine tests that need to be done in the next 24 hours is also generated.

The 24-hour fluid input cycle starts at 9 a.m. This time was chosen for the convenience of the junior medical staff. If any part of the previous 24-hour's fluids were not given, they are noted and discarded.

At 2 p.m. a 10-ml aliquot of the urine output is sent to the laboratory for estimation of the urea and electrolyte content. The result of this test is made available by the next morning to estimate the excretion of nitrogen and electrolytes as detailed above.

At 5 p.m. the results of the preceding 24-hour blood and urine tests are obtained from the laboratories. These are entered into the computer for the accurate calculations of the balances used to generate the balance tables and graphs.

In summary, the fluid input 24-hour period starts and ends at 9 a.m., whilst the fluid output period starts and ends at 6 a.m. The houseman enters information into the computer twice each day, at 8 a.m. to obtain the following day's requirements and at 5 p.m. to input the previous day's results. The time needed to enter these results into the computer is no more than ten minutes each day. This is a great saving in the effort spent by the house surgeon compared to the manual method of calculating the patient's inputs, outputs and balances.

The Program

The program runs on any IBM-compatible microcomputer. It will run best on a double floppy or hard disc colour system with a minimum of 128 K of RAM, as each of the program and the data need 64 K of memory to run. On a single floppy system, a minimum of 512 K is needed. This is because the system has to be configured to include a RAM disc of 360 K capacity, leaving over 128 K of memory for use by the program and data. The program is loaded into the RAM disc and the floppy drive is freed for use by the data disc. A colour system is needed if the graphs and tables are to be displayed in colour. The flow chart of the program is shown in Fig. 10.2.

On loading the program the user is greeted with the welcome screen which reminds him to place the data disc into disc drive (A:). The program then obtains the date directly from the computer if it is equipped with an internal clock/calendar or requests the user to enter the date. The main menu is then displayed. This allows the user the following alternatives: entering a new patient into the program; monitoring a previously entered patient; changing the program parameters; exiting out of the program. Each of these options will now be described.

Entering a New Patient into the Program

On selection of this option the user is able to enter a new patient into the TPN program. First, the user must satisfy the computer that the patient does indeed require parenteral feeding. To determine this the computer asks the user if the patient has a functional gastro-intestinal tract; if a negative answer is given the computer is satisfied that TPN is indicated. If the computer is told that the patient has a functional gastro-intestinal tract, a summary of the various types of enteral feeding (oral, nasogastric, gastrostomy, jejunostomy) is displayed and

6 a.m.

End of 24 hour fluid collection
Each output is weighed and charted
Start of next 24 hour fluid collection

8 a.m.

Data entered into computer

Total fluid input.
Total fluid output.
Urea & electrolyte content of urine
(based on previous day's spot test)

Print-out obtained from computer

Next 24 hour's requirements
Laboratory request form
Pharmacy request form

Blood tests recommended by computer taken

Solutions recommended by computer written

9 a.m.

Any fluids not gone through
are discarded
New regimen is commenced

2 p.m.

10 ml urine sent to laboratory
for analysis of :

Na content
K content
Urea content

5 p.m.

Results entered into computer

Blood test results
Accurate fluid input
Accurate fluid output
Accurate U&E output

Fig. 10.2. Flow chart of program for computerised total parenteral nutrition.

1. Hospital number
2. Title
3. First name
4. Surname
5. Consultant in charge of case.
6. Diagnosis
7. Ward
8. Present weight in Kg
9. Height in Cm
10. Age
11. Average temperature over last 24 hours
12. Fluid output over last 24 hours
13. Sodium output over last 24 hours
14. Potassium output over last 24 hours

Fig. 10.3. Data needed to enter a new patient into the total parenteral nutrition program.

the user is asked if there is a reason why one of these is not suitable. The patient can only be entered into the TPN program by stating that none of the enteral methods is suitable.

Having satisfied the computer that TPN is indicated, the patient's details have to be entered. Fig. 10.3 lists these details. When these have been entered the computer checks if the patient's weight is in the correct range for his height using the body mass index and informs the user if the patient is underweight, overweight or normal weight for his height. The body mass index is the weight in kilograms divided by the square of the height in metres, and the normal range is 20 to 23. The program then requests information on any factors that may increase the nutritional requirements (Fig. 10.4). If the required factor is not included then by using the last option, the clinician can enter a user-defined stress factor. The program then calculates the calorie, nitrogen, sodium, potassium and fluid requirements of the patient.

0. No stress   Stress factor = 1.00

1. Surgery   Stress factor = 1.25

2. Major surgery   Stress factor = 1.50

3. Major trauma   Stress factor = 1.40

4. Burns under 30%   Stress factor = 1.50

5. Burns 30% – 50%   Stress factor = 1.70

6. Burns 50% – 70%   Stress factor = 1.90

7. User defined   Stress factor = x.xx

Fig. 10.4. Factors increasing the nutritrional requirements.

Calculation of Calorie Requirements

The basal energy requirement is taken as being the same as the resting energy expenditure (REE) calculated by the Harris–Benedict [7] equations. These equations are:

for the male, $REE = 66.432 + (13.751 \times W) + (5.003 \times H) - (6.775 \times A)$

for the female, $REE = 655.095 + (9.653 \times W) + (1.849 \times H) - (4.675 \times A)$

where REE is resting energy expenditure, W is weight (kg), H is height (m) and A is age (years)

The equations are weighted for each of the following factors: pyrexia (10 % for each degree centigrade above 37°C); underweight (10 % for each 10 % below ideal weight); selected stress factor.

Calculation of the Nitrogen Requirements

The nitrogen requirement is taken as 250 milligrams per kilogram of body weight and then adjusted so that the calorie : nitrogen ratio falls into the required range. The range used in the program is 180 to 220 but this can be altered by the user if necessary.

Calculation of the Fluid and Electrolyte Requirements

These are calculated by adding the net losses of each in the previous 24 hours to the normal daily requirements. Some authorities use the serum values of the electrolytes in the calculation of the requirements, but we elected not to do so in order to make the program more usable; it must be possible to predict the following day's requirements with unknown serum values.

The results of these calculations are then displayed on the screen along with the calorie nitrogen : ratio (Fig. 10.5). Any of the values can be altered if required leaving ultimate control of the prescription to the clinician. If any of the altered values lie outside normal limits a warning message is displayed on the screen and the clinician then has the opportunity to modify the value or ignore the warning.

If the nitrogen requirement of the patient is less than 12 grams per day the computer asks if the anticipated period of feeding is less than two weeks; if the answer is positive then the computer selects peripheral vein feeding instead of central TPN. This can be accepted or rejected by the clinician. The computer displays the regimens available (Fig. 10.6) and selects the one that has the closest fit to the patient's requirements. The regimens used by the program are based on the standard solutions provided by Travenol. These can be given on their own or with 500ml of 10 % or 20 % Intralipid solution – nine possible combinations. A tenth option is a standard three-litre solution for PVN. The clinician may agree with the computer's choice or substitute one of the other regimens. The computer then displays the additives also required over the next 24-hour period. These, along with the blood and urine tests needed that day, are automatically printed. It is our policy to use a low-nitrogen solution with no Intralipid for the first 48 hours of feeding, and the program's selection of fluids for infusion during this initial period takes account of this. The clinician is then asked to provide

HERE ARE THE CALCULATED REQUIREMENTS OF THIS PATIENT

1. Total calorie   requirement : 2933 Kcal.

2. Total nitrogen   requirement : 14.0 Grams.

3. Total sodium   requirement : 90   Meqs.

4. Total potassium requirement : 70   Meqs.

5. Total fluid   requirement : 2800 Mls.

The Kcal/Nitrogen ratio = 210

Fig. 10.5. Calculated requirements for a patient on total parenteral nutrition.

AVAILABLE FEEDING SOLUTIONS

PARENTERAL NUTRITION   PERIF. NUT.

	(LOW NITROGEN)			(MEDIUM NITROGEN)			(HIGH NITROGEN)			PERIF. STAND. SOL.	CALC. REQ.
	NO LIPID	W/10% LIPID	W/20% LIPID	NO LIPID	W/10% LIPID	W/20% LIPID	NO LIPID	W/10% LIPID	W/20% LIPID		
Kcal	1800	2900	3800	1800	2900	3800	1800	2900	3800	1800	2933
Nit	9.4	9.4	9.4	14.3	14.3	14.3	20.3	20.3	20.3	10.0	14.0
Cal/N	190	308	408	125	202	265	90	142	187	180	210
Vol	2500	3000	3000	2500	3000	3000	3000	3500	3500	3000	6055
Reg No	1	2	3	4	5	6	7	8	9	10	

THE MOST APPROPRIATE REGIMEN FOR THIS PATIENT IS REGIMEN NO : 5

DO YOU WISH TO ACCEPT THIS REGIMEN (Y/N) ?

Fig. 10.6. Available feeding solutions.

information on the TPN line used (see later) and this concludes the entry of a
new patient into the program.

Monitoring a Previously Entered Patient

When this option is selected, the computer displays the names and hospital
numbers of all the patients previously entered on the data disc. The user is asked
to select the patient he wishes to monitor by entering the appropriate hospital
number. The main details of that patient: name, hospital number, age, ward and
diagnosis are displayed for confirmation that the correct patient has been
selected. When this has been confirmed, the TPN monitoring menu (Fig. 10.7) is
displayed. Each option on this menu will be discussed in turn.

Entering the Patient's Blood Results

On selecting this option a submenu is displayed which allows the user to select
among entering the haematology, biochemistry and bacteriology blood results.
For each of these a grid is displayed with the blood parameters horizontally and
the last seven days' results vertically. By selecting the result to be entered, its
value, and the date the test was taken, results can be entered anywhere on the
grid. There is full error-checking on the values entered to reduce input errors,

```
        ┌──────────────────────────────────────┐
        │     T.P.N. MONITORING MENU           │
        └──────────────────────────────────────┘

   1. Enter Blood, Weight and Temperature Results.

   2. Enter Fluid Input and Output Results.

   3. Calculate Next 24 Hour's Requirements.

   4. Print and Display Balances in Table Form.

   5. Print and Display Balances and Blood Results in Graph Form.

   6. Enter T.P.N. Line Database.

   7. Exit to Main Menu.

                  PLEASE ENTER CHOICE :
```

Fig. 10.7. Total parenteral nutrition monitoring menu.

and any results that lie outside the normal limits are high-lighted in red. A separate routine allows input of the patient's daily weight and temperature.

Entering the Fluid Input and Output of the Patient

On selection of this option the user is able to enter the fluid input and output of the patient over each 24-hour period. To enter the fluid input the computer displays a selection of intravenous fluids available (Fig. 10.8) and by selecting the number of the fluid and the volume given the computer automatically calculates the cumulative volume, electrolyte, nitrogen and calorie content of the infused fluids. If the fluid transfused does not appear on the list, the computer requests information on the contents of that fluid. Once all the infused fluids over a 24-hour period have been entered the data are automatically entered into the TPN transactions database.

To enter the fluid output of a patient, the screen displays the possible outputs: urine, vomit, drains, fistulae and others. The appropriate outputs are selected in turn and the volume and electrolyte content of each one is entered. If the electrolyte content is not known the computer will use default values. In the case of urine, the user is also asked to enter its urea and protein content. Once all the outputs over a 24-hour period have been entered the computer calculates the total nitrogen, electrolyte and fluid output for that 24-hour period. It then obtains the input of those substances from the TPN transactions database held

---

J. Smith   First Day of TPN = 10/2/1987   Today = 22/2/1987   FLUID INPUT

FLUID INPUT ROUTINE

1. Low Nitrogen
2. Medium Nitrogen
3. High Nitrogen
4. Perifusin
5. 10% Intralipid
6. 20% Intralipid
7. 10% Dextrose
8. 20% Dextrose
9. Normal Saline
10. Normal Saline + 20 Kcl
11. Normal Saline + 40 Kcl

12. Dextrose Saline
13. Dextrose Saline + 20 Kcl
14. Dextrose Saline + 40 Kcl
15. 5% Dextrose
16. 5% Dextrose + 20 Kcl
17. 5% Dextrose + 40 Kcl
18. Hartman's Solution
19. P.P.F.
20. Oral Fluids
21. Other 1
22. Other 2

23. Select this option when all the inputed fluids have been entered

PLEASE SELECT THE NUMBER OF THE FLUID YOU WISH TO ENTER :

Fig. 10.8. Fluid input of patient on total parenteral nutrition.

on the data disc for the same 24-hour period, calculates the balances and updates the TPN transaction database. The nitrogen output (per 24-hour period in grams) is calculated by adding the nitrogen loss as urinary urea, urinary protein, retained urea and non urinary nitrogen. The formulae for calculating these are derived as follows:

1. Nitrogen loss due to urinary urea:

    Each molecule of urea contains two atoms of nitrogen. The molecular weight of nitrogen = 14.

    Therefore each Mol of urea contains $2 \times 14 = 28$ g of nitrogen. Therefore each mMol of urea contains 0.028 g of nitrogen.

    The non-urea nitrogen of the urine (other than proteinuria) is assumed to be ⅕ that of urea.

    Then the total urinary nitrogen = (0.028 × mMol urea) + ((0.028 × mMol urea)/5).

    Therefore the total urinary nitrogen = mMol urea/30 g of nitrogen.

2. Nitrogen loss due to retained urea:

    The distribution volume of urea in the body is approximately 60 %.

    Therefore each mMol rise of the plasma urea = 0.028 × (60/100 × weight) = 0.016 × weight

    Therefore the retained urea nitrogen (in g) = (body weight in kg × rise in plasma urea in mMol/l)/60

3. Nitrogen loss due to proteinuria:

    On average one gram of nitrogen is contained in each 6.25 g of protein.

    Therefore nitrogen loss due to proteinuria (g) = proteinuria/6.25

4. Non-urinary nitrogen losses (mostly faeces and sweat):

    Due to the impracticalities of collecting these substances, the nitrogen loss is estimated rather than collected.

    Faecal and sweat nitrogen losses estimated at 1.5 g.

Calculating the Daily Requirements of the Patient

Once the fluid input, fluid output, weight, temperature and blood results over a 24-hour period have been entered, by selecting option 3 on the monitoring menu (Fig. 10.7), the fluid, calorie, nitrogen, electrolyte and vitamin requirements for the following 24-hour period are calculated. If this option is selected before entering all the results needed for the calculations, the program alerts the user and returns back to the monitoring menu. The calculations for the following 24-hour period are done with the same formulae described for entering a new patient into the program. As before, a hard copy listing the solutions, additives, blood and urine tests required for this period is automatically printed. The program keeps track of the date and thus its recommendations of blood tests and additives are based on this to accommodate for tests and additives that are not needed daily.

A laboratory request form for the urine and blood tests recommended is also automatically printed out. This reduces the work-load of the junior doctors. It also helps the laboratories to identify the samples of patients on TPN so that the tests can be carried out urgently.

Displaying the Balances in Table Form

A patient on TPN can only be managed effectively if trends can be spotted early. It is very important to be able to view the inputs, outputs and balances of the patients in a clear accurate manner, and this is where the advantages of computerised as compared to manual monitoring really become apparent. The inputs, outputs and balances of nitrogen, sodium, potassium and fluid can be viewed for each 7-day period in the form of a table by selection of option 4 from the monitoring menu. The user can scroll up and down this table and thus view the balances of the whole period of time that the patient has been on TPN. If required a hard copy can also be obtained of this table. On the screen the positive balances appear in blue and the negative ones in red for instant recognition of positive or negative balance for each of the substances.

Displaying the Balances in Graphical Form

Trends can be more easily spotted if the representation of the inputs, outputs and balances are displayed graphically. This is made possible by option 5 in the main menu. The user is first asked which period of TPN he wishes to be displayed, from as short as a 3-day to as long as a 100-day period. The user is then asked to select which graph he wishes to view, the options being sodium, potassium, nitrogen, fluid balance or all together. He can then view graphically the input, output and balance of the factors selected. The input and output are depicted as line graphs with the balance as a bar graph; each of these graphs can also be printed out if required. The graphs are automatically scaled for minimum and maximum values. Fig. 10.9 shows a dot matrix output of the nitrogen graph for a 14-day period. If all the graphs are to be viewed together, only the balances are displayed without the input and output in order to avoid crowding. The dot matrix output of this is shown in Fig. 10.10.

TPN Line Database

This is the final option on the monitoring menu (Fig. 10.7), and by using this option details of the TPN line are entered. The items that can be entered are:

1. Type of line
2. Route inserted (cutdown, stab, subclavian, jugular)
3. Name of surgeon
4. Grade of surgeon (HS, SHO, registrar, senior registrar, consultant)
5. Time taken for insertion
6. Date inserted
7. Date removed

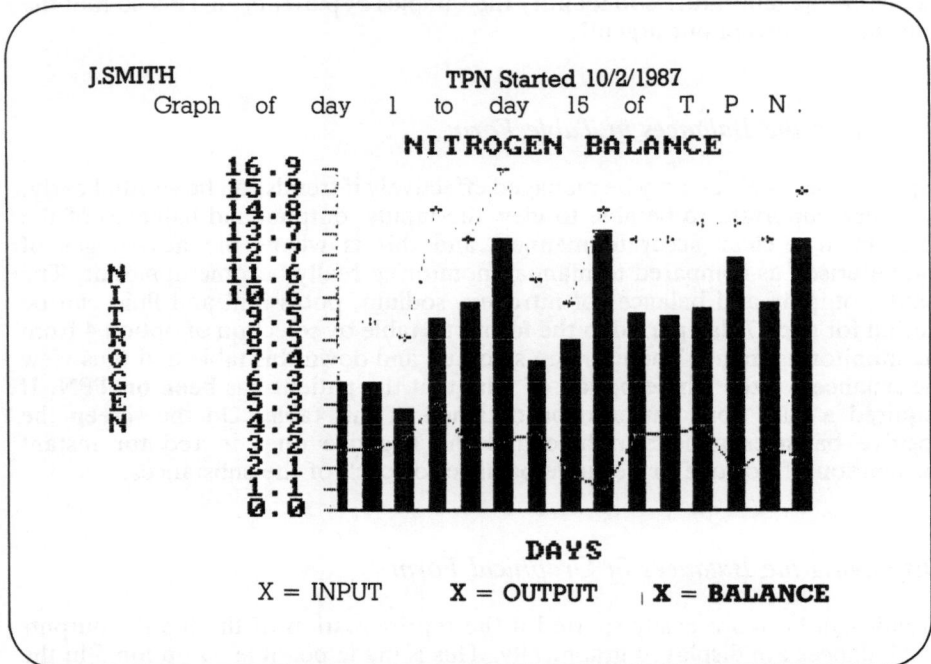

Fig. 10.9. Printout of the nitrogen input, output and balance for a 14-day period.

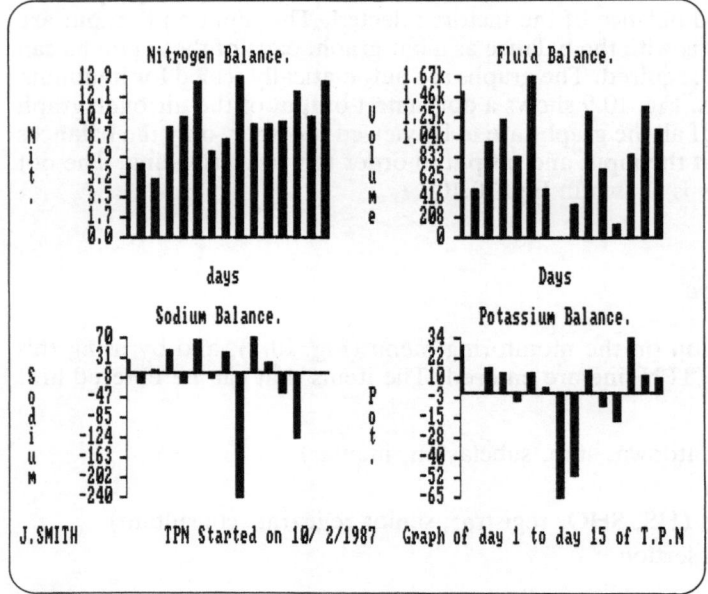

Fig. 10.10. Dot matrix nitrogen, fluid, sodium and potassium balances for a 14-day period.

8. Reason removed (sepsis, blocked, TPN ended)
9. Comment

These details can be entered for a maximum of three separate TPN lines, but it is possible to record the number of lines used if this exceeds three. This provides a very useful database of TPN lines and their complications. This database is stored on disc in standard ASCII form and may be used for audit purposes.

Patient Progress Report

This part of the program is being written at the moment. On selection of this option it will be possible to obtain a summary of the progress of TPN with details of when TPN was started, for how many days the patient has been fed, how successful it has been, and any complications that have occurred. It is planned to produce a similar summary at the conclusion of TPN.

Changing the Program Parameters

This is the maintenance part of the program. It allows the entry of details of the hospital and the personal preferences of the physician using the system. These include:

1. Name of the hospital to be included in the printed reports
2. Calorie : nitrogen ratio to be used in the program
3. Selection between standard pre-mixed TPN solutions or a prescription to pharmacy for mixing the solutions on a daily basis.
4. If standard pre-mixed TPN solutions are to be used, entry of details of the available TPN solutions in the hospital.
5. Desired frequency of blood tests and additives.

This option is also used to prepare the data disc for use by the TPN program.

Leaving the Program

This option closes all the data files, saves the updated versions on the data disc and returns the user to the operating system of the computer.

Future Developments

The program described is a means of reducing the junior doctors' administrative work-load, eliminating errors of calculation and helping with the selection of regimens for patients on TPN. Apart from error checking on blood results entered and warnings of an inappropriate calorie : nitrogen balance of the suggested fluids there is little assistance given by the program for dealing with problem patients.

Renal Failure and Diabetes. At present the program is only appropriate for adults who are metabolically stable and who do not suffer from renal failure or diabetes. One of our aims in the future is to incorporate additional modules to make it possible for the program to manage the TPN requirements of patients suffering from these conditions. The program will have to be able to recognise the existence or development of these conditions either from the diagnosis entered at the start of TPN or from the results of the blood tests entered during monitoring. On recognition of such a patient the program will automatically bring into action the new modules needed to manage the patient more appropriately.

Patient Selection Module. Another weakness in the program is the patient selection module. This at present has two screens. The first displays a summary of the various enteral and parenteral methods of feeding when a new patient is to be entered into the program. The second screen is displayed if it is declared that the patient has a functional gastro-intestinal tract. It displays a summary of the enteral feeding methods available and suggests feeding the patient by one of these methods. We are planning to enlarge the patient selection module and place it after the entry of the patient details so that suggestions of enteral nutrition are by-passed if an absolute indication for TPN has been entered as the patient's diagnosis. Similarly if a diagnosis where TPN is not usually indicated is entered, then a suitable method of enteral nutrition will be strongly recommended along with a suitable regimen based on the patient's calculated requirements. We are planning a question-and-answer module to determine the most appropriate method of feeding, when the patient's diagnosis does not indicate it.

Monitoring Success of Feeding. The patient's response to the nutrition provided is currently measured only by the nitrogen balance and daily weight. Weight gain may in fact be a misleading guide to the success of TPN as it may only reflect salt and water retention. This may be deduced by looking at the patient's fluid and electrolytes balance graphs. We wish to incorporate a module that will do this automatically, alert the clinician and take appropriate action. Monitoring the patient's progress by nitrogen balance is probably not enough and we will be incorporating additional anthropometric measurements such as mid-arm circumference, triceps skin thickness as well as other methods such as the grip test and the serum protein estimations.

Rationalising the Tests Required. The program suggests the blood and urine tests required based on a predetermined frequency. For example a full blood count and serum urea and electrolytes measurements are recommended daily, liver function tests are recommended every other day, while clotting studies are recommended weekly. This is appropriate for the average patient at the start of TPN but may not be so for a patient that has been on TPN for a month and has been completely stable on it. In order to be able to tailor the tests needed to the patient's condition the program must be able to make an assessment of the patient's progress. The way we propose to achieve this is by analysing the trends of the nitrogen, fluid and electrolyte balances as well as trends of the blood parameters.

Help Screens. We plan to incorporate help screens into the program. By hitting a special key the user will be able to interrupt the program at any time and display the help screen related to that part of the program. We hope this will make the program more educational as we shall include details of the formulae used and the thinking behind the program.

Database Facilities. The auditing facilities of the program are limited at present to producing databases in standard ASCII format on the data disc. There is no interrogation facility of these databases. They can be interrogated by any off-the-shelf database package that can read standard ASCII files. We hope to incorporate simple reporting facilities in the near future mainly on the TPN line database giving line sepsis rates related to the type of catheter used, route of insertion and time taken to insert it, and giving the name of the surgeon.

The disadvantage of incorporating all these facilities into the program is that it will become cumbersome to use, because many additional menus will be required to select the new features. Another disadvantage is that the program will be too big to fit on a floppy disc and will require more of the computer's memory especially if used in a single floppy system where the program has to be loaded into the RAM disc. Some of these facilities may be completely unnecessary for some institutions such as small district general hospital where TPN is only used occasionally. To accommodate the different needs of the users we plan for the standard program to consist of only the features mentioned in the previous section. To this basic program the user will be able to install any number of the enhancements planned and thus have a program best suited to his needs. The modular approach of PASCAL makes this intention particularly easy to implement.

Discussion

This project started off with a small program written in BASIC which calculated the energy and calorie requirement of a patient. Since then it has grown into a much bigger program, made possible by abandoning BASIC and changing to PASCAL. Without the structured programming discipline of PASCAL we do not feel it would have been possible to develop this program in the relatively easy manner and in the short time it has taken.

We have been using this program in our hospital since the middle of 1986 and the junior medical staff in charge of the patients on TPN have found it is practical as well as pleasurable to use. It takes about half an hour to teach a person how to use the program fully.

We compared computerised TPN with the manual charts we had been using earlier. We did this by entering the information from charts of patients managed manually into the program. We discovered a multitude of errors, some simple mathematical ones, others due to omissions such as entering the volume of saline given in addition to the three-litre-bag solution but not including its electrolyte content. In many cases the balance charts were not done because of the shortage of time. In the patient's case-notes details of the TPN lines used were not complete. These observations confirm that computerisation of TPN has a very definite advantage even if it is used solely for data collection and for approaching TPN in an organised and disciplined manner.

Computers have been very slow in making an impact on the medical profession. There are many areas of medicine where the application of computers can be of invaluable help. We hope that in this chapter we have described such an application.

References

1 James RM, Roberts JM, Harvey PW, Bellis JD, Cooper RI (1978) A computerised scheme for the preparation of parenteral nutrition regimes. Med Inf (Lond) 3: 77–86
2 Goggin MJ (1979) The use of a small programmable calculator in intravenous feeding. Med Inf (Lond) 4: 115–118
3 Goggin MJ, Hoskins HT (1985) Management of parenteral nutrition aided by microcomputer. Med Inf (Lond) 10: 5–12
4 Anthony NG, Cyril Wong SK (1985) A microcomputer program for parenteral nutrition. Br J Parenter Ther [May]: 63–67
5 Colley CM, Fleck A, Howard JP (1985) Pocket computers: a new aid to nutritional support. Br Med J 290: 1403–1406
6 Skaredoff MN, Consoli P (1985) Iperalimentazione. A program to calculate hyperalimentation needs. Int J Clin Monit Comput 1: 245–249
7 Harris JA, Benedict TG (1919) Biometric studies of basal metabolism in man. Carnegie Institute of Washington, publication no. 279

11 Computer-Simulated Medical Emergencies: Teaching Programs for Undergraduate Education

P.R. Edwards, J.R. Coughlan, M.J. Taylor and W.A. Corbett

Introduction

Medical education has always demanded a great deal from the medical student who has to acquire numerous skills and retain a vast amount of information on a diverse number of subjects during both the preclinical and the clinical periods. The number of subjects is increasing as is the depth to which each must be taught in order for the student to gain a satisfactory understanding.

It is essential for the student to be both interested and motivated as the process of acquiring such vast amounts of data is often tedious and demoralising, and any attempt to improve the learning process must be of interest to both the student and the teacher. A variety of teaching techniques have been introduced into many medical schools over the past decade in an attempt to provide stimulating and enjoyable alternatives to sitting down with a book. The techniques have not all been fully evaluated and the inclusion of many is often due to the department concerned having a specific interest. The provision of a number of complementary techniques within a single department could be of great benefit to the student as it is unlikely that any one single teaching technique could provide a fully comprehensive basis for medical instruction. Clinical education, however, has a good basic teaching system. It has correctly relied upon tuition at the bed-side where the student is able to elicit from patients their symptoms, to discover the signs of specific diseases, and to observe and discuss investigation and treatment. As this situation obviously necessitates student and patient interaction it should allow the student to develop skills of patient communication. Thus, bed-side tuition provides the foundation which may be supplemented by a variety of teaching techniques and aids. Techniques currently used to expand upon facts acquired at the bed-side include seminars, lectures, study groups, audio-visual aids and private study. Many, or all, may be used within a subject and the exact role that each technique will play depends upon many factors including subject matter, teacher preferences and financial limitations.

Audio-visual aids range from films and videos to slides and computer-based displays. The introduction of these aids has been made possible by the major technological advances which have occurred over the past two to three decades and they now provide a number of stimulating alternatives to the more traditional techniques. In conjunction with this new technology, although not necessarily as a result of it, educational philosophy has changed and it is now considered that the student should be more actively involved in the learning process. It might be reasonably assumed that passive procedures such as lectures and seminars will diminish in importance whereas techniques involving self-tuition and active participation will be promoted.

Interaction between patient and student is an extremely important reason why bed-side teaching will always be considered to be the major form of undergraduate clinical instruction. However, the interaction is always passive as the student observes the treatment of a patient undertaken by others. This situation is eminently understandable as obviously it would be unacceptable for the patient to be managed by unqualified staff. This limitation does mean that students are unable to learn by testing their ideas or thoughts on patient management and so have lost an opportunity to learn by their mistakes. Teaching methods have been designed and developed in order to overcome some of these particular shortcomings. The introduction of computer technology to teaching practices has provided a flexible technique which is becoming increasingly accessible to students of all specialties. In medical practice microcomputers may serve many functions including clinical audits, discharge and clinic letters and, in a few centres, they have been used to assist in the diagnosis of patients with abdominal pain [1]. Surprisingly, the wide availability of such microcomputers has not led to their general acceptance by the majority of physicians. This reluctance seemingly originates from the initial difficulties encountered with the early machines, particularly as the computer seemed to represent all that was bad in technologically advanced machinery. The particular factors which gave rise to this situation were the necessity to learn a new language both to program the machine and to converse with the computer specialist, and the lack of good objective evaluation of the programs which had been written for the medical educational field [2]. These factors have resulted in a distinct lack of user friendliness and have ensured that some clinicians have avoided computers altogether and so computers in medical education, although available for a considerable time, have yet to find their place.

Teaching Programs

Early programs were written on main-frame computers and so were restricted to major teaching centres. The programs were complex and required dedicated programmers to write them. Inevitably, the programmers were as interested in the capabilities of the machine as in the improvement in the student.

Early Simulation

Computers used as teaching aids in medicine have often been programmed to simulate the patient and although there are obvious limitations on the extent of their realism they do seem to have a frontal role in medical education. The early simulations simply represented the patient as a set of symptoms, signs and laboratory values and students were required to interrogate the computer in order to try to build up a clinical picture from which they were expected to make a diagnosis. One of these early programs was based on a data matrix of the percentage prevalence of fifty symptoms in six specific diseases [3]. As each student commenced the program the computer randomly selected one of the diseases and generated a random two-figure number. This number was compared to the percentage values for each symptom and sign. If the latter value was greater than the randomly generated number the computer recognised this as a symptom or sign demonstrated by the patient and subsequently informed the student when interrogated. A list of symptoms and signs recognised by the computer was required by the student before the program could be run. All that was then required of the student was to type in the symptom they desired to know about and they were then informed by the computer simply whether or not the patient had that symptom. On progression through the program the student was requested to construct a symptom complex and then decide on a diagnosis. If incorrect, a tutoring sequence was initiated which selected the symptom most appropriate to the correct diagnosis. Assessment of the program was not undertaken although its applications and possible benefits were appreciated.

Static Simulation

Over a decade later, in 1976, Murray [4] described a program consisting of a set of nine management problems all of which might be commonly encountered in general practice. Each problem required the student to make a number of management decisions by utilising a grading system. As each decision point arrived a set of options were provided for the student who then graded each with regard to its importance in the correct management of the patient. The grades allocated to each option were then compared by the computer to grades previously allocated by eleven experts and if found to be outside previously agreed ranges the students were asked to reconsider their answers. Background information on the patient was not provided within the program but was contained in a separate booklet which became an integral part of the simulation. Furthermore, the program was considered to be merely an offshoot of the book enquiring of the student the answers to a set of questions and then "marking" them, providing immediate assessment as in the case of a simple multiple-choice questionnaire booklet. Further criticisms of the program noted its inflexibility as the student was not allowed to interrogate the program and answers given were independent of each other, so that mistakes made at one level were not cumulative [5]. Regrettably the program was not assessed for the ability to influence the learning performance of the students.

Dynamic Simulation

Simulations have been developed which more realistically depict the management of a patient by allowing the patient's condition to change both with time and in response to the treatment initiated. Programs based on dynamic simulations may be subdivided into two categories [6], those where there is true mathematical simulation and those with pseudosimulation.

True Mathematical Simulation

The patient is represented as a mathematical equation which is solved by the computer as each variable is changed. These programs are difficult to produce because biological systems are difficult to represent in mathematical form when a large number of variables are considered under a multiplicity of conditions. One of the least involved programs was described by Geddes et al. [7] and concerned the response of patients to drugs used in the treatment of epilepsy. This program utilised a simple pharmaceutical model to calculate the blood level of the drug from which the response to treatment and occurrence of side-effects was estimated. A suitable patient was generated by the computer which had been programmed to provide patients of different ages and weights with one of four types of epilepsy. The student was required to select the drug of choice and its dose in each patient. Inappropriate medication, due to an incorrect choice of either drug or dose immediately resulted in the computer giving an error message. On receipt of one of these the user had to reconsider the management policy and either select a different drug or modify the prescribed dose. Once the correct treatment is given, the program allows the patient to be followed up in the out-patient department at regular intervals where modification of the treatment regime may have to be undertaken in the light of further developments in the disease process.

More complex mathematical simulations have been developed including the treatment of diabetic ketoacidosis, maintenance of fluid and electrolyte balance and a cardiovascular-pulmonary model in which the computer program can be used to simulate diseases such as myocardial infarction, pulmonary embolus and arterial or venous bleeding [8].

Pseudosimulation

Pseudosimulations are a form of dynamic simulation in which discrete decision points exist and where alternative pathways are followed depending upon the students' management decisions. These programs are easier to write than the mathematical simulations but still represent the real-life situation quite accurately. In 1982, Dugdale [9] described a program in which the principal features were that the patient's condition was not only altered by the appropriate treatment but also changed with time. Simulated time was incorporated into the program such that each investigation or procedure was allocated a time value which was incremented as each was undertaken. As simulated time progressed the patient's condition invariably deteriorated unless specific resuscitative measures were performed. The program allowed a certain degree of flexibility, the student being able to commence initial resuscitation, progress to the information gathering and subsequently return to continue resuscitation. Computer-student interaction was limited because a book had to accompany the program. The book included a brief history of the patient and a list of questions on the history, examination and investigations; each reply had a serial number which the computer had been programmed to recognise and to respond to with a comment about the presence of the symptom or sign or result of the investigation. This level of interaction means that the students merely type in a number and so have less stimulation to think about the problem as all of the symptoms and signs are already documented for them.

Higher levels of interaction have been developed where the student is not only required to consider the questions that should be asked but also to try and determine exactly which questions the computer will recognise. This higher form of interaction is known as free-text input and provides a stimulating and demanding form of student-computer interaction. However, this is still quite primitive as the computer recognises key words and a few basic syntactical relations. The computer may be made to appear to respond appropriately even though it failed to "read" a number of words from the question posed.

A variety of programs is available with a wide range of levels of interaction, computer assistance and subjects depicted. Few of these programs are available outside their respective medical schools and institutions and experience in their use has been limited to the students of specific schools only. Similarly few programs have been fully evaluated with regard to improving problem-solving skills. The lack of evaluation of many programs has led some physicians to conclude that although they may be new and technologically advanced they are no more effective than a pencil and paper or a book. A recent report [10] suggested that computer-based education, in general, may "be an improvement over more conventional educational and evaluative methods". Thirty-two studies were considered in the report which concluded that the time to complete a course of study may be shortened by computer-based education. The report detailed greater efficiency in learner functioning and improved problem-solving skills in 80 % of the studies reviewed. The improved efficiency was considered to be due to the facility which allowed the students to progress at their own paces whilst receiving continuous feedback on their individual performances. The question of cost savings was not satisfactorily answered by the studies reviewed and it was certainly considered that in this respect further work was required.

Certain factors were clearly important in this particular aspect, particularly the role the computer was allocated in each subject. The principal area in which computer-based instruction was considered to be able, potentially, to provide a financially rewarding technique was when frequent repetition of the teaching sessions was required particularly over an extended period of time. In medical education a great deal more work is required to determine the exact role for the computer and as yet few studies have objectively considered this question.

Clinical Scenario

The aim of our study was to develop two dynamic computer simulations and to evaluate these with regard to the acquisition of factual material. The subjects chosen for simulation were two patients who had been managed by the authors over the preceding eighteen months and both represented problems associated with major blood loss. One patient had been stabbed in the right side of his abdomen whilst awaiting his customary Saturday night post-lager diet of fish and chips and represented the problem of occult blood loss. The second patient presented with a haematemesis and melaena secondary to oesophageal varices and obviously represented a problem of overt blood loss.

We chose to utilise a BBC model B microcomputer on which to develop the simulations as this machine has a wide usage and a suitable authoring system was also available. The authoring system, Microtext, was designed to provide a simple programming package allowing users with an interest in computers to develop their own programs [11]. Although relatively simple to use, Microtext offers the facility to recognise words and phrases which permits a natural interactive dialogue between user and program so that the students can type directly into the keyboard the treatment or investigation they wish to be performed. In addition, Microtext has particularly attractive features including a facility to incorporate the BBC's graphics and sound commands. The graphics facilities allowed the production of simple line-diagrams of clinical and endoscopic findings, representations of abdominal examination findings and chest X-ray signs (Fig. 11.1a,b). As the chest X-ray was represented graphically a facility was provided whereby students could interrogate the computer for an interpretation of the signs shown if they had not fully understood the diagram (Fig. 11.2). The sound facilities have been used to add a little light-hearted distraction to the simulations although the user is allowed to enjoy a silent program if so desired. The musical accompaniment ranges from a simulated ambulance siren in the introduction to an electrical "Congratulations" or "The Death March" at the end depending on the outcome.

The simulations considered the management of the two patients throughout their in-patient stays and so included the initial resuscitation and investigative procedures, the definitive surgical treatment and the associated complications which developed. Using this basis we divided the simulations into three levels. The student has to negotiate each level successfully before progressing to the next.

At the start of each simulation the program includes an introductory module describing the format of the program and explaining the keyboard and particularly the keys relevant to the simulation. Subsequent comments detail the presenting symptoms of the patient and describe the clinical scene. The student is given the role of the surgical registrar on call.

Both patients are admitted via the Accident and Emergency Department and are reasonably well on arrival, but this situation does not continue for long as their conditions deteriorate rapidly as simulation time progresses. During this first stage the student is expected to acquire a history, perform an examination and commence resuscitative procedures. The options available in the program are concerned with these specific points although a number of further choices are also available. The options within the program may be considered as

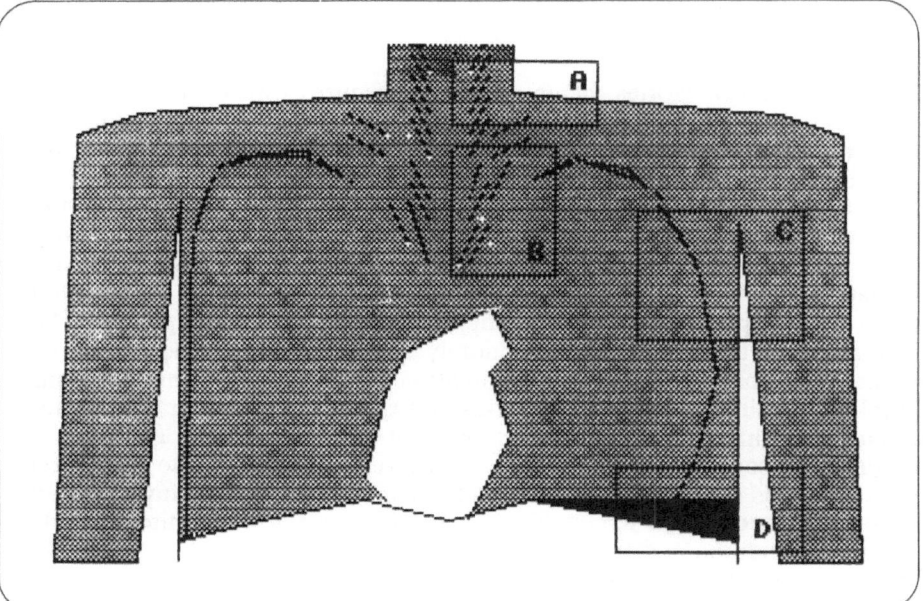

Fig. 11.1a,b. Simple line-diagrams of findings on examination of patient.

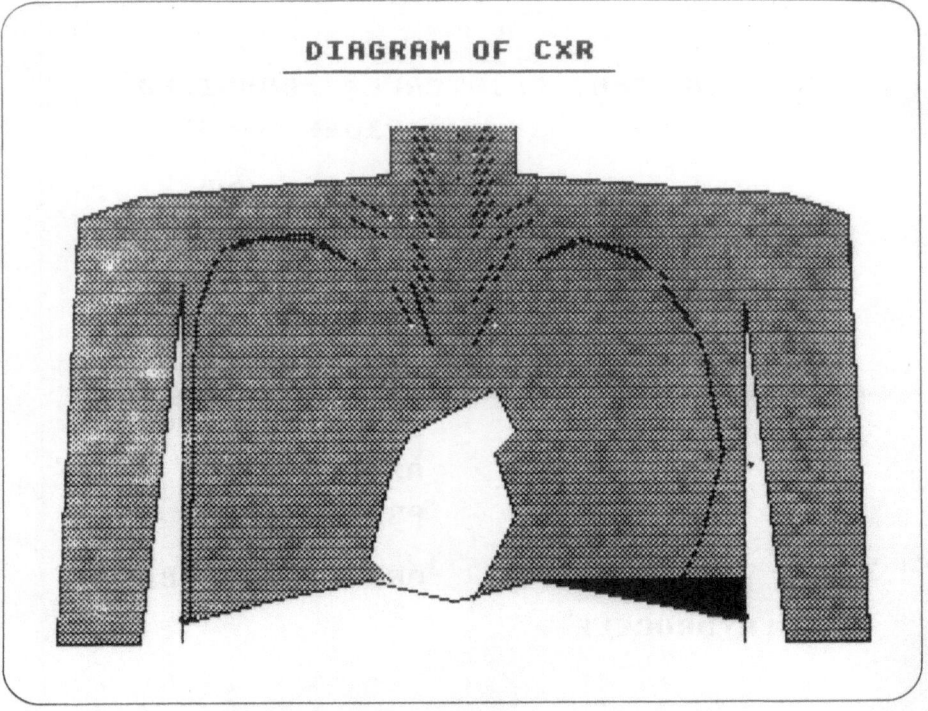

Fig. 11.2. Computer interpretation of chest X-ray.

representing three categories, namely those procedures which are essential to the correct management of the patient, those which may supplement the treatment of the patient but which are not essential and, thirdly, those which are not beneficial and will waste time.

Each option within the first level is allocated a time value representing the average time to perform the procedure in a typical hospital in an emergency situation. As the student progresses through the program selecting particular investigations and treatment schedules the time allocated to each is incremented on a clock in the program so emphasising the time spent with the patient. The initial time on the clock is generated randomly by the computer at the start of the program. As a history is taken, examination performed and investigations undertaken the simulated time progresses and the patient's condition deteriorates although this inexorable decline may be reversed by the appropriate treatment. The condition of the patient is reflected in the pulse rate and blood pressure which is continually updated at the completion of each investigation and is documented on the screen. The student is then able to monitor directly the patient's condition and the effect the treatment is having.

The screen display used in the programs is divided into three parts, Fig. 11.3. Each part is used for detailing specific areas of interest with regard to the patient's management. The upper third of the screen is reserved for the patient's details which include the name, cardiovascular parameters and results of the

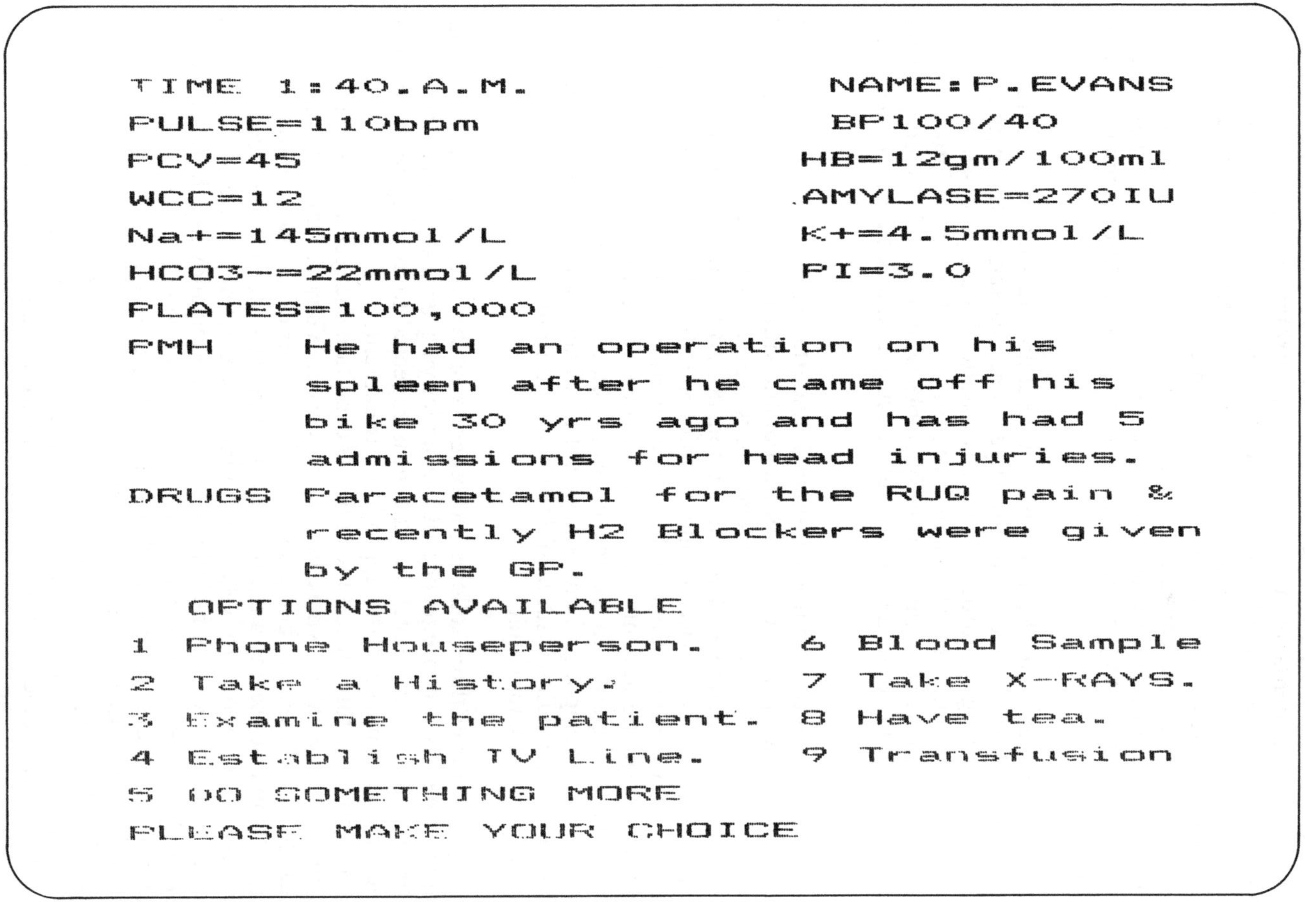

```
TIME 1:40.A.M.           NAME:P.EVANS
PULSE=110bpm             BP100/40
PCV=45                   HB=12gm/100ml
WCC=12                   AMYLASE=270IU
Na+=145mmol/L            K+=4.5mmol/L
HCO3-=22mmol/L           PI=3.0
PLATES=100,000

FMH  He had an operation on his
     spleen after he came off his
     bike 30 yrs ago and has had 5
     admissions for head injuries.

DRUGS Paracetamol for the RUQ pain &
      recently H2 Blockers were given
      by the GP.

     OPTIONS AVAILABLE

1 Phone Houseperson.      6 Blood Sample
2 Take a History.         7 Take X-RAYS.
3 Examine the patient.    8 Have tea.
4 Establish IV Line.      9 Transfusion
5 DO SOMETHING MORE

PLEASE MAKE YOUR CHOICE
```

Fig. 11.3. Screen display of program.

haematological and biochemical investigations undertaken. The simulated time is also detailed in this part of the screen. The middle third of the screen is reserved for comments about the investigations undertaken or treatment planned. These may detail problems encountered whilst undertaking the procedure, or possible sequelae of them, or the comments may detail the findings of the investigations. The lower third of the screen, in the case of the menu-driven simulation, contains a menu of options available to the student at that point in the program. In the free-text input mode, this part of the screen is reserved for students to type in requests or to receive helpful comments about their choice.

Level One. To negotiate the first level successfully the student is required to obtain a history and to examine, investigate and resuscitate the patient. The student may not progress through to level two until all these processes have been performed successfully. Furthermore, progress cannot be made into level two unless the patient is also physiologically stable with a systolic blood pressure greater then one hundred millimetres of mercury and a pulse rate of less than one hundred.

Level Two. In level two definitive therapy is undertaken. For the trauma patient this necessitates a laparotomy and for the patient with an upper gastro-intestinal bleed this requires a diagnostic endoscopy (Fig. 11.4) and progression to endoscopic sclerotherapy or balloon tamponade. At this point the students are able to call upon the services of more senior members of the team or, if they wish, they may continue alone and "try their hand" at the procedures required. During this stage the students are required to make decisions such as the incision to be used for laparotomy or the pressure required for the inflation of the balloon during oesophageal tamponade with a Sengstaken–Blakemore tube. If the surgical intervention is successful the patient is returned either to the ward or to the intensive therapy unit.

Level Three. Level three follows the progress of the patient as complications develop either as a consequence of the underlying disease process or of the treatment given. In this level the student is expected to investigate the patient further and to commence the appropriate treatment.

Throughout the three levels the patient's condition changes and of course may deteriorate to the extent where death may ensue. Whatever the outcome, be it successful with the patient being discharged home, or otherwise, the students are given the choice of seeing a chronological summary of their chosen options and they may also choose to view an optimum treatment schedule. Microtext includes as one of its many facilities a summary option allowing all the decisions made by the student to be recalled and listed. This allows teaching to take place around the computer keyboard when the selections and decisions made by the student can be discussed and suitable algorithms may be considered and criticised. More simply it provides an opportunity for self-criticism whereby the student may, on reflection, realise where the mistakes were made. Further assistance is given in level three with the provision of a number of references for the interested student. At completion of the program, therefore, the student may choose either to view the above details or to return to the start and to begin the simulation again.

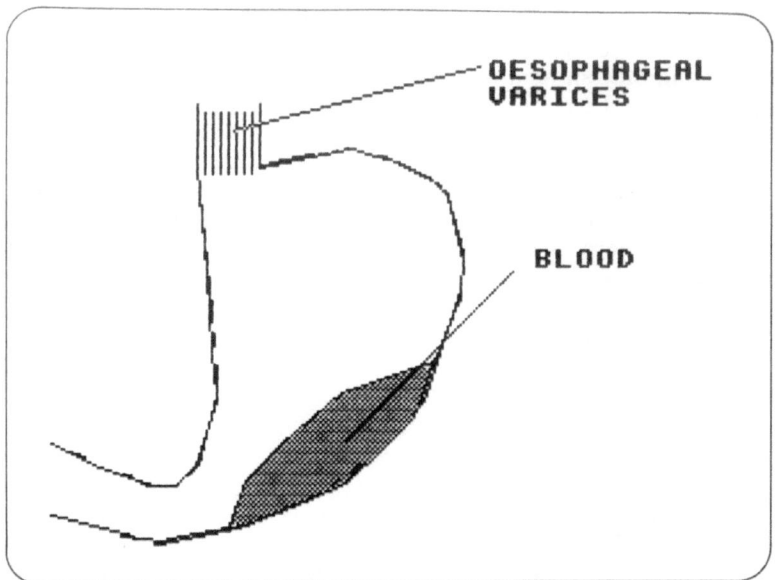

Fig. 11.4.   Screen display of diagnostic endoscopy.

Testing

We have now been able to test these programs on clinical students and have generally been impressed with the feedback we have received. Initially we asked for comments about the general format and presentation, the presence of any bugs and the difficulties with operation. Although the comments received were varied, many were directed at a small number of specific points.

In one simulation the information and the comments on the investigations and treatments were presented instantaneously whilst the other scrolled the data onto the screen. The difference, surprisingly, was commented upon by a large percentage of initial users who, almost without exception, favoured the instantaneous presentation. All students were offered the choice of either a menu-driven or free-text-input simulation although the majority opted for the easier of the two; the menu-driven format.

Educational Trial

After an initial trial period during which the difficulties were ironed out the programs were evaluated by testing for the improvement in the retention of factual material by students. The performance of the students was assessed by multiple choice questionnaire (MCQ). Fifty-two students were invited to undertake the study: they were all in the third year of medical school, corresponding with their first year of clinical training. Clinical experience and knowledge was limited and they were all in their first surgical attachment at the time of the study. The students had already been randomly divided into three groups for teaching purposes and these groups were retained for the study. The evaluation of the computer simulations was undertaken over a 1-week period. At the commencement and completion of the study the students were required to sit an MCQ examination related to the topics in the simulations.

Following the initial MCQ Group One students received a tutorial on the topics and were subsequently allowed free access to the computer programs during the normal working hours of the next seven days. No extra tuition was given around the computers. The students of Group Two received the same tutorial but were not allowed access to the computers. Group Three students received no formal teaching on the topics discussed in the simulations until the second MCQ had been completed.

Results

During the study week Group One students were expected to run the simulations during their spare periods and they were not expected to forego their normal studies and duties. Each student was asked to note the time spent on each simulation. At the end of the study week all students sat a second MCQ. Both MCQs were answered anonymously and marked negatively and each had a maximum mark of fifty. The time spent on each simulation varied greatly and it was obvious that some students had run the simulations a number of times. Overall more time was spent on the trauma program which we thought reflected the content of the program in that it was both more detailed and used free-text input, rather than the quicker and less demanding menu-driven format.

The results of the MCQ examinations are shown in Table 11.1. Statistical analysis was performed by the Student's t-test. There is no statistical difference between the initial scores of all three groups. The final scores of both Group One and Group Two were significantly better than their initial scores, whereas Group Three showed no significant improvement on their initial result. Although both Group One and Group Two improved, Group One demonstrated a significantly greater improvement than Group Two. We concluded from these results that tutorials improve a student's knowledge as determined by the MCQ but that computer simulations in conjunction with a tutorial are more effective than a tutorial alone in assisting the student to retain factual information.

Conclusion

Microtext as an authoring system proved to be versatile and relatively simple in use. The facilities within the system and on the BBC microcomputer allowed stimulating and educational programs to be developed. The potential role of such programs may be as alternatives to text-books particularly when the student may have short periods of spare time which otherwise are often wasted.

Although the authoring system proved to be relatively simple to use the time spent in developing these programs was considerable. A number of people contributed to the simulations including both surgeons and computer scientists and it would be difficult to estimate the exact time spent by an individual on the

Table 11.1. Results of multiple choice question examinations

	No. of students	Scores		d	Significance
		Start	1 week		
Group 1	20	7.9	19.25	+11.35	$P<0.001$
Group 2	16	4.5	12.9	+8.4	$P<0.01$
Group 3	16	7.1	10.3	+3.2	Not significant

project. As a conservative estimate we think at least six hundred man-hours were spent on developing the two programs but considerably less time would be required for any subsequent ones, assuming that a similar format was retained.

For the future it might be feasible for groups from various centres to be involved in the production of a library of such simulations once a basic format had been agreed upon. Similarly cooperation between centres may enable the role of such programs to be defined and their efficacy in improving medical training to be determined.

References

1 De Dombal FT, Leaper DJ, Horrocks JC, Staniland JR, McCann AP (1974) Human and computer-aided diagnosis of abdominal pain: further report with emphasis on performance of clinicians. Br Med J 1: 376–380
2 Schwartz MW, Hanson CW (1982) Microcomputers and computer based instruction. J Med Educ 57: 303–307
3 Entwisle G, Entwisle DR (1963) The use of a digital computer as a teaching machine. J Med Educ 38: 803–812
4 Murray TS, Cupples RW, Barber JH, Hannay DR, Scott DB (1976) Computer assisted learning in undergraduate medical teaching. Lancet 1: 474–476
5 Simpson MA (1976) Computer assisted learning. Lancet 1: 859
6 Hoffer EP, Barnett GO, Farquhar BB, Prather PA (1975) Computer aided instruction in medicine. Annu Rev Biophy Bioeng 4: 103–117
7 Geddes C, Kendle KE, Selkirk AB, Walker W (1983) KEKEPI: A computer program for simulating the therapeutic responses of patients suffering from idiopathic epilepsy. Med Educ 17: 325–330
8 Dickinson CI (1977) A computer model of human respiration. MIP Press Ltd, Lancaster, England
9 Dugdale AE, Chandler D, Best G (1982) Teaching the management of medical emergencies using an interactive computer terminal. Med Educ 16: 27–30
10 Computer technology in medical education and assessment (1979) (US) Office of Technology Assessment, Washington, DC
11 Bevan E, Watson R (1983) Microtext for the BBC Microcomputer. Acornsoft Ltd, Cambridge

Subject Index